PEJMAN HAJBABAIE

Understanding High Blood Pressure

First edition

This book was professionally typeset on Reedsy.
Find out more at reedsy.com

Contents

1

Chapter 1: Understanding Hypertension

Definition and Importance of Blood Pressure

Blood pressure is the force exerted by circulating blood on the walls of blood vessels. It is typically expressed in millimetres of mercury (mmHg) and is recorded with two numbers: systolic pressure, the higher number, measures the pressure in arteries when the heart beats, while diastolic pressure, the lower number, measures the pressure in arteries between heartbeats. Understanding these values is crucial, as they reflect the state of cardiovascular health and the efficiency of the circulatory system.

The importance of monitoring blood pressure cannot be overstated, particularly in the context of hypertension, which affects millions worldwide. High blood pressure is often termed the 'silent killer' because it frequently presents no symptoms, yet it can lead to severe health complications, including heart disease, stroke, and kidney failure. Regular monitoring allows individuals to recognise potential issues early and take necessary actions to manage their blood pressure effectively.

Dietary approaches play a significant role in managing blood pressure. Consuming a balanced diet rich in fruits, vegetables, whole grains, and low-fat dairy products, while reducing sodium intake, can significantly lower blood pressure levels. Additionally, understanding the impact of specific dietary components, such as potassium and magnesium, can empower individuals to make informed choices that contribute to better cardiovascular health.

Physical activity is another critical factor in blood pressure management. Engaging in regular exercise strengthens the heart, improves blood circulation, and can reduce systolic and diastolic pressures. Incorporating activities like walking, cycling, or swimming into daily routines not only aids in weight control but also enhances overall physical and mental well-being, thereby reducing the risk of hypertension.

Lastly, psychological factors, including stress and anxiety, are closely linked to blood pressure changes. Chronic stress can lead to behaviours that exacerbate hypertension, such as poor eating habits and inactivity. Therefore, adopting stress management techniques, such as mindfulness, meditation, or regular physical activity, is essential for maintaining healthy blood pressure levels, especially for older adults and those at risk of hypertension-related complications.

Types of Hypertension - Essential vs. Secondary

Hypertension, commonly referred to as high blood pressure, is categorised into two main types: essential hypertension and secondary hypertension. Essential hypertension, which accounts for the majority of hypertension cases, does not have a specific identifiable cause. Instead, it is influenced by a combination of genetic, environmental, and lifestyle factors. This type of hypertension often develops gradually over many years and can be exacerbated by factors such as poor diet, lack of physical activity, and stress, making it a significant concern for public health.

In contrast, secondary hypertension is caused by an underlying medical condition. This type of hypertension can arise from various factors, including kidney disease, hormonal disorders, or the use of certain medications. Unlike essential hypertension, secondary hypertension can often be treated by addressing the underlying issue, which may lead to a reduction in blood pressure. Understanding the distinction between these two types is crucial for effective management and treatment strategies.

Dietary approaches play a significant role in managing both types of hypertension. For individuals with essential hypertension, adopting a heart-healthy diet that emphasises fruits, vegetables, whole grains, and lean proteins can lead to substantial improvements in blood pressure. Additionally, reducing sodium intake and limiting processed foods are vital steps to consider. For those with secondary hypertension, dietary modifications may be essential in conjunction with treating the primary condition.

Physical activity is another critical component in managing hypertension. Regular exercise can help lower blood pressure and improve overall cardiovascular health. Individuals with essential hypertension are often encouraged to engage in aerobic exercises, such as walking or cycling, while those with secondary hypertension may need to tailor their exercise regimen based on their specific medical condition. Understanding the impact of physical activity on blood pressure regulation is important for everyone, regardless of the type of hypertension they may have.

Lastly, psychological factors, including stress and anxiety, can significantly affect blood pressure levels. Stress management techniques, such as mindfulness and relaxation exercises, can be beneficial for individuals with essential hypertension, while those with secondary hypertension may need to address the psychological implications of their underlying health issues. Recognising the interplay between psychological factors and hypertension is essential for a comprehensive approach to managing high blood pressure effectively.

Causes and Risk Factors

High blood pressure, or hypertension, is a multifaceted condition influenced by a variety of causes and risk factors. Genetics plays a significant role, as individuals with a family history of hypertension are more likely to develop the condition themselves. This hereditary aspect highlights the importance of understanding one's family medical history when assessing personal risk. Furthermore, age is another critical factor, with the likelihood of developing hypertension increasing as one grows older, particularly in individuals over the age of 45.

Symptoms and Diagnosis of Essential Hypertension

Essential hypertension, often referred to as primary hypertension, is a condition characterised by consistently elevated blood pressure without any identifiable cause. Many individuals with essential hypertension may not experience noticeable symptoms, which is why this condition is frequently termed a 'silent killer.' Over time, however, high blood pressure can lead to significant health issues, including heart disease, stroke, and kidney damage. Understanding the symptoms, or lack thereof, is crucial for early detection and management of this prevalent condition.

While many individuals may not exhibit overt symptoms, some may experience vague signs such as headaches, dizziness, or shortness of breath during physical exertion. These symptoms can often be mistaken for other health issues, which complicates the diagnosis of essential hypertension. Regular monitoring of blood pressure is essential, especially for those who have risk factors such as obesity, a sedentary lifestyle, or a family history of hypertension. Awareness of these risk factors can prompt individuals to seek medical advice even in the absence of clear symptoms.

Diagnosis of essential hypertension typically begins with a comprehensive medical history and a physical examination, followed by multiple blood pressure readings taken on different occasions. Blood pressure is classified into categories ranging from normal to stage 2 hypertension, and accurate measurement is critical for establishing a diagnosis. In some cases, healthcare professionals may recommend additional tests, such as blood tests or electrocardiograms, to assess any potential complications arising from prolonged high blood pressure.

Lifestyle factors play a significant role in both the development and management of essential hypertension. Dietary approaches, including reducing salt intake and increasing potassium-rich foods, are often advised as part of a comprehensive management strategy. Furthermore, engaging in regular physical activity can help lower blood pressure and improve overall cardiovascular health. Psychological factors, such as stress and anxiety, can also exacerbate hypertension, highlighting the importance of a holistic approach to treatment.

In conclusion, while essential hypertension may not present obvious symptoms, its implications for long-term health are profound. Regular monitoring and a proactive approach to lifestyle modifications are essential for managing this condition effectively. For older adults, understanding the risks associated with hypertension and the importance of routine check-ups can significantly impact their quality of life. By recognising the subtle signs and maintaining open communication with healthcare providers, individuals can take charge of their health and mitigate the risks linked to essential hypertension.

Symptoms and Diagnosis of Secondary Hypertension

Secondary hypertension is a type of high blood pressure that occurs due to an identifiable underlying condition. Unlike primary hypertension, which develops gradually over many years, secondary hypertension can appear suddenly and can often be attributed to specific health issues. Common causes include kidney disease, hormonal disorders, and certain medications. Recognising the symptoms associated with secondary hypertension is crucial for timely diagnosis and treatment, as addressing the underlying cause can significantly improve the patient's condition.

Patients with secondary hypertension may experience a range of symptoms, some of which may be subtle or easily overlooked. Headaches, particularly those that are severe or frequent, are commonly reported. Other symptoms can include shortness of breath, fatigue, and visual changes. In some cases, individuals may not exhibit any symptoms at all, making regular blood pressure checks essential for early detection. Understanding these symptoms can help individuals seek medical advice promptly and potentially prevent complications.

Diagnosis of secondary hypertension involves a comprehensive assessment that includes a detailed medical history and physical examination. Healthcare providers often perform blood and urine tests to check for underlying conditions such as kidney dysfunction or hormonal imbalances. Imaging studies, such as ultrasound or CT scans, may also be utilised to identify structural abnormalities. By determining the root cause of hypertension, healthcare professionals can tailor treatment strategies effectively, leading to better outcomes for patients.

In addition to standard diagnostic procedures, lifestyle factors play a significant role in managing secondary hypertension. A thorough evaluation of dietary habits, physical activity levels, and psychological stressors is essential. For instance, excessive salt intake and obesity can exacerbate hypertension, while regular physical activity can help lower blood pressure. Understanding the interrelationship between these factors can empower individuals to take proactive steps in managing their health and mitigating the effects of hypertension.

Overall, recognising the symptoms and undergoing appropriate diagnostic procedures for secondary hypertension is vital for effective management. With the right approach, including lifestyle modifications and medical interventions, individuals can significantly improve their blood pressure levels and overall health. It is important for everyone, especially those at risk, to stay informed about hypertension and its implications, facilitating timely action and better health outcomes.

When to Suspect Secondary Hypertension?

Secondary hypertension is often overlooked in the assessment of high blood pressure. It is essential to consider this condition when standard treatment methods fail to yield the expected results. Unlike primary hypertension, which is generally idiopathic, secondary hypertension has identifiable causes that can significantly influence blood pressure levels. Understanding when to suspect secondary hypertension is crucial for appropriate diagnosis and management, especially in individuals who present with sudden or severe hypertension.

Certain clinical indicators should raise suspicion for secondary hypertension. These include a sudden onset of high blood pressure in an individual with previously normal readings, resistant hypertension that does not respond to conventional treatment, or hypertension occurring at a younger age than typical. Additionally, the presence of specific symptoms such as headaches, visual disturbances, or episodes of sweating may indicate an underlying condition contributing to the elevated blood pressure. Recognising these signs can prompt further investigation into potential causes.

Common conditions associated with secondary hypertension include renal disease, endocrine disorders, and certain medications. For instance, conditions such as chronic kidney disease can lead to fluid retention and subsequent increases in blood pressure. Endocrine disorders, such as hyperaldosteronism or Cushing's syndrome, can also disrupt the body's regulatory mechanisms for blood pressure. It is vital for healthcare providers to take a thorough medical history and consider these conditions during the evaluation process.

Lifestyle factors play a role in both primary and secondary hypertension. However, when hypertension is secondary, addressing the root cause can lead to significant improvement in blood pressure control. For example, if a patient is found to have obstructive sleep apnoea, treating this condition may alleviate the hypertension. Additionally, psychological factors, such as stress and anxiety, can exacerbate blood pressure issues, complicating the clinical picture. Thus, a holistic approach to treatment that considers both physiological and psychological elements is essential.

Monitoring and follow-up are critical in managing patients suspected of having secondary hypertension. Regular blood pressure checks, along with appropriate diagnostic tests, can help in identifying the underlying cause. Once diagnosed, tailored treatment strategies can be developed, potentially incorporating lifestyle modifications, medication adjustments, or referrals to specialists. By being vigilant and proactive, healthcare providers can significantly improve outcomes for patients affected by secondary hypertension.

Management Differences Between the Two

Management of high blood pressure can differ significantly between various approaches, each tailored to meet individual patient needs and circumstances. These strategies encompass lifestyle modifications, pharmacological interventions, and complementary therapies. Understanding these differences is crucial for effective hypertension management, particularly when considering patient age, existing health conditions, and personal preferences.

Dietary approaches play a pivotal role in managing hypertension. The DASH diet, rich in fruits, vegetables, whole grains, and low-fat dairy, is widely recommended for its efficacy in lowering blood pressure. Additionally, reducing sodium intake is crucial, as high salt consumption can exacerbate hypertension. Tailoring dietary recommendations to individual tastes and cultural preferences can enhance adherence and improve outcomes.

Physical activity is another cornerstone of hypertension management, with evidence supporting its role in lowering blood pressure and improving overall cardiovascular health. Regular exercise, such as brisk walking, cycling, or swimming, can have both immediate and long-term benefits. The management plan should consider the patient's physical capabilities, preferences, and any comorbid conditions that may influence exercise choices.

Psychological factors also play a significant role in hypertension management. Stress and anxiety can contribute to elevated blood pressure, making it essential to address these aspects within treatment plans. Techniques such as mindfulness, cognitive behavioural therapy, and relaxation exercises can be beneficial. Understanding the psychological components of hypertension can lead to a more holistic approach to management.

Lastly, the type of medication prescribed for hypertension can vary based on individual patient profiles. There are several classes of antihypertensive medications, each with distinct mechanisms and potential side effects. Regular monitoring and adjustments may be necessary to find the most effective regimen. Effective communication between healthcare providers and patients about these differences is vital for optimal management of hypertension.

Complications of Untreated Hypertension

Hypertension, often termed the silent killer, can lead to a myriad of complications when left untreated. The cardiovascular system is particularly vulnerable, with untreated high blood pressure significantly increasing the risk of heart disease and stroke. Over time, the increased pressure on the artery walls can cause them to thicken and harden, a condition known as atherosclerosis. This not only impairs blood flow but also heightens the risk of heart attacks and other serious cardiovascular events.

One of the most concerning complications of untreated hypertension is its effect on the kidneys. The kidneys play a crucial role in regulating blood pressure and filtering waste products from the blood. Chronic high blood pressure can damage the blood vessels in the kidneys, leading to kidney disease or even kidney failure. This can necessitate dialysis or a kidney transplant, significantly impacting an individual's quality of life and overall health.

Moreover, untreated hypertension can adversely affect the brain, leading to cognitive decline and an increased risk of dementia. The blood vessels that supply the brain can become damaged, reducing blood flow and resulting in a condition known as vascular dementia. Additionally, strokes can occur due to blood clots or bleeding in the brain, both of which are exacerbated by high blood pressure. The neurological consequences can be devastating, affecting memory, mobility, and overall functioning.

The eyes are not spared from the effects of uncontrolled hypertension either. Hypertensive retinopathy is a condition where high blood pressure damages the blood vessels in the retina, potentially leading to vision loss. Regular eye examinations can help identify changes in the retina early, allowing for timely intervention. However, if left unchecked, the complications can lead to irreversible damage and blindness.

Finally, untreated hypertension can also impact mental health, contributing to anxiety and depression. The stress of managing a chronic condition, coupled with the fear of potential complications, can create a cycle of emotional distress. Addressing both the physical and psychological aspects of hypertension is essential for comprehensive management, underscoring the importance of a holistic approach in understanding and treating this prevalent condition.

2

Chapter 2: Dietary Approaches to Managing Hypertension

The DASH Diet: Principles and Benefits

The DASH diet, or Dietary Approaches to Stop Hypertension, is a dietary plan specifically designed to combat high blood pressure. It focuses on consuming a balanced diet rich in fruits, vegetables, whole grains, and lean proteins while reducing the intake of saturated fats, cholesterol, and sodium. By emphasising nutrient-rich foods, the DASH diet aims to provide essential vitamins and minerals that support heart health and overall well-being.

One of the key principles of the DASH diet is its emphasis on lowering sodium intake. Research has shown that reducing sodium can lead to significant decreases in blood pressure levels. The diet recommends limiting sodium to no more than 2,300 milligrams per day, with an ideal goal of 1,500 milligrams for individuals with hypertension. This reduction can be achieved by avoiding processed foods, reading labels carefully, and opting for fresh ingredients whenever possible.

In addition to sodium reduction, the DASH diet encourages an increase in potassium-rich foods. Foods such as bananas, spinach, and sweet potatoes are not only delicious but also help to balance the effects of sodium in the body. Potassium is essential for maintaining healthy blood pressure levels, making it a crucial component of the DASH diet. The diet also promotes the consumption of low-fat dairy products, which provide calcium and vitamin D, both known to support cardiovascular health.

The benefits of the DASH diet extend beyond blood pressure control. Studies have indicated that individuals who adhere to this dietary plan may experience weight loss, improved cholesterol levels, and reduced risk of heart disease. Additionally, the DASH diet's focus on whole foods rather than processed options can lead to better overall health and well-being. This holistic approach makes it not just a diet, but a sustainable lifestyle change.

Incorporating the DASH diet into daily life can also be complemented by physical activity, which is vital for managing hypertension. Regular exercise, alongside dietary changes, can enhance the effectiveness of the DASH approach. Furthermore, addressing psychological factors such as stress management is equally important in the comprehensive management of hypertension. Together, these principles form a robust framework for understanding and controlling high blood pressure, making the DASH diet a valuable tool in the fight against hypertension.

Sodium Intake and Blood Pressure

Sodium intake plays a significant role in regulating blood pressure levels, making it a critical focus for those aiming to manage hypertension. The body requires sodium to function properly, but excessive consumption can lead to fluid retention, which in turn increases blood volume and elevates blood pressure. Current dietary guidelines recommend limiting sodium intake to reduce the risk of hypertension and its associated complications. By understanding the relationship between sodium and blood pressure, individuals can make informed dietary choices that support their overall health.

Many processed and packaged foods contain high levels of sodium, often exceeding the recommended daily limits without individuals realising it. This hidden sodium can contribute to a cumulative intake that may lead to hypertension over time. Reading food labels and selecting fresh, whole foods can significantly reduce sodium consumption. Incorporating fruits, vegetables, and lean proteins not only enhances nutrition but also helps maintain healthier blood pressure levels.

Research indicates that even a modest reduction in sodium intake can lead to noticeable improvements in blood pressure for many individuals. For instance, a decrease of just 1,500 mg of sodium per day can result in significant drops in blood pressure, particularly for those already experiencing hypertension. In addition to dietary changes, increasing physical activity can further amplify these benefits, creating a comprehensive approach to blood pressure management that combines both diet and exercise.

Furthermore, it is essential to consider the psychological factors that may influence dietary choices and sodium intake. Stress, for example, can lead to unhealthy eating habits, including the consumption of high-sodium foods. By addressing stress through relaxation techniques, mindfulness, and physical activity, individuals may find it easier to stick to a low-sodium diet and improve their blood pressure control. Understanding these connections can empower individuals to take charge of their health more effectively.

In conclusion, sodium intake is a crucial aspect of managing blood pressure and preventing hypertension. By being mindful of sodium consumption and making healthier dietary choices, individuals can significantly impact their blood pressure levels. Moreover, combining dietary approaches with physical activity and stress management can offer a holistic strategy for better health outcomes. As awareness of the importance of sodium in our diets grows, so does the potential for improved cardiovascular health and overall well-being.

Foods to Embrace and Avoid

Maintaining a balanced diet is crucial for managing high blood pressure, and understanding which foods to embrace and avoid can significantly impact overall health. Foods rich in potassium, such as bananas, oranges, and leafy greens, can help balance sodium levels in the body, thereby aiding in blood pressure control. Incorporating whole grains, lean proteins, and healthy fats like those found in nuts and avocados is also beneficial, as they provide essential nutrients without contributing to hypertension.

On the other hand, certain foods should be avoided to maintain optimal blood pressure levels. Processed foods often contain high levels of sodium, which can lead to increased blood pressure. Items such as canned soups, deli meats, and frozen dinners should be consumed sparingly. Additionally, sugary beverages and excessive alcohol intake can contribute to weight gain and elevated blood pressure, making it essential to limit their consumption in one's diet.

Incorporating a variety of fruits and vegetables not only enhances flavour but also provides vital vitamins and minerals that support heart health. Berries, for instance, are rich in antioxidants and have been linked to lower blood pressure. Similarly, beets contain nitrates, which can help dilate blood vessels and improve blood flow. Thus, increasing the intake of these foods can complement other lifestyle changes aimed at managing hypertension.

Another aspect to consider is the timing and method of food preparation. Cooking methods such as steaming, grilling, or baking are preferable to frying, as they retain the nutrients without adding unhealthy fats. Preparing meals at home allows for better control over ingredients, helping to avoid hidden sugars and salts often found in restaurant dishes and takeaways.

Lastly, maintaining a healthy weight through balanced nutrition and regular physical activity is essential for hypertension management. Engaging in exercise can enhance the effectiveness of dietary approaches, reducing stress and promoting overall heart health. By understanding the relationship between diet and blood pressure, individuals can make informed choices that contribute to long-term wellness.

Meal Planning and Preparation Tips

Meal planning is a crucial aspect of managing high blood pressure, as what we eat directly influences our cardiovascular health. To begin, individuals should focus on incorporating a variety of fruits and vegetables into their diets, aiming for at least five servings each day. These food groups are rich in essential nutrients and antioxidants, which can help lower blood pressure and improve overall health. Planning meals around these key ingredients not only enhances flavour but also adds vital nutrients that are beneficial for hypertension management.

Another important tip is to choose whole grains over refined grains. Whole grains such as brown rice, quinoa, and whole grain bread are packed with fibre and nutrients that support heart health. When meal planning, consider creating a list of whole grain options and incorporating them into daily meals. This simple switch can contribute to better blood pressure control while providing sustained energy throughout the day.

It is equally important to limit sodium intake, as excessive salt consumption is a significant contributor to high blood pressure. When preparing meals, opt for herbs and spices to enhance flavour instead of salt. Reading food labels and selecting low-sodium products can make a substantial difference in your diet. Preparing meals at home allows for greater control over ingredients, which is essential for those looking to manage their hypertension effectively.

Incorporating lean proteins into meal plans is another strategy that supports blood pressure management. Options like skinless poultry, fish, legumes, and low-fat dairy products provide necessary protein without the saturated fats found in red meats. By planning meals that include these healthier protein sources, individuals can help maintain a healthy weight and reduce the risk of hypertension-related complications.

Lastly, staying organised and prepared can make meal planning a more manageable task. Setting aside time each week to plan meals, create shopping lists, and prepare foods in advance can alleviate the stress of last-minute cooking. This proactive approach not only helps in maintaining a balanced diet but also fosters a healthier lifestyle overall, which is essential for those managing high blood pressure.

3

Chapter 3: The Role of Physical Activity in Blood Pressure Control

Understanding Physical Activity Guidelines

Understanding physical activity guidelines is essential for managing high blood pressure effectively. Regular physical activity plays a significant role in lowering blood pressure and improving overall cardiovascular health. The guidelines suggest a combination of aerobic exercises and strength training to maximise the benefits. Engaging in moderate-intensity activities such as brisk walking, cycling, or swimming for at least 150 minutes a week is recommended for adults.

For those with hypertension, it is crucial to tailor physical activity to individual needs and capabilities. Starting with low-impact exercises can help those who are new to fitness or have health concerns. Gradually increasing the intensity and duration of workouts can lead to better results without overwhelming the individual. Consulting healthcare professionals before beginning a new exercise regimen is advisable, especially for older adults and those with existing health conditions.

Incorporating physical activity into daily routines can be an effective strategy for managing blood pressure. Simple changes, such as taking the stairs instead of the lift or walking during lunch breaks, can significantly contribute to achieving the recommended activity levels. Additionally, group activities or classes can provide social support and motivation, making exercise more enjoyable and sustainable.

It's essential to consider the psychological aspects of physical activity as well. Engaging in regular exercise can reduce stress levels and improve mental well-being, which are both beneficial for blood pressure management. Mindful practices such as yoga or tai chi can also be included in the exercise regimen, offering both physical and mental health benefits.

Finally, monitoring the effects of physical activity on blood pressure is vital. Keeping track of progress through regular check-ups and self-monitoring can help individuals stay motivated and make necessary adjustments to their routines. Overall, understanding and adhering to physical activity guidelines can play a pivotal role in controlling hypertension and promoting a healthier lifestyle.

Types of Exercises Beneficial for Hypertension

Hypertension, or high blood pressure, can be managed effectively through various types of exercises that promote cardiovascular health and overall well-being. Aerobic exercises, such as walking, jogging, cycling, and swimming, are particularly beneficial as they increase heart rate and improve blood circulation. Engaging in these activities for at least 150 minutes a week can lead to significant reductions in blood pressure levels. Additionally, aerobic exercises help in maintaining a healthy weight, which is crucial for individuals managing hypertension.

Strength training also plays an essential role in controlling blood pressure. Incorporating resistance exercises, such as weight lifting or body-weight workouts, at least twice a week can enhance muscle strength and metabolic rate. This type of exercise not only aids in weight management but also contributes to improved insulin sensitivity, which is linked to better blood pressure regulation. It is important for individuals to focus on proper technique and form to prevent injuries while performing strength training exercises.

Flexibility and balance exercises, including yoga and tai chi, can provide additional benefits for those with hypertension. These activities not only promote relaxation and reduce stress but also improve overall body function and mobility. Studies have shown that mind-body exercises like yoga can lower blood pressure by enhancing mindfulness and reducing the physiological effects of stress. Practising these exercises regularly can contribute to a holistic approach to managing hypertension.

For older adults, low-impact exercises such as walking or water aerobics are advisable, as they are gentler on the joints while still providing cardiovascular benefits. Engaging in regular physical activity can help combat the risks associated with hypertension in this age group, including heart disease and stroke. Additionally, social interactions during group exercises can improve mental health, which is often an overlooked aspect of hypertension management in older populations.

Incorporating a variety of exercises into one's routine can yield the best results in managing hypertension. It is essential to consult with healthcare professionals before starting any new exercise programme, especially for those with existing health conditions. By choosing enjoyable activities and maintaining consistency, individuals can effectively lower their blood pressure and enhance their quality of life, ultimately leading to better health outcomes for those affected by hypertension.

The Impact of Regular Exercise on Blood Pressure

Regular exercise has been shown to have a significant impact on blood pressure levels, making it a vital component of hypertension management. Engaging in physical activity helps to improve heart function and vascular health, which are crucial for maintaining optimal blood pressure. Studies indicate that both aerobic and resistance training can lead to reductions in systolic and diastolic blood pressure, benefiting individuals across various age groups and fitness levels.

The physiological mechanisms behind the blood pressure-lowering effects of exercise are multifaceted. Physical activity promotes better blood flow, reduces arterial stiffness, and enhances the body's ability to regulate blood pressure through the release of certain hormones. Additionally, regular exercise can help with weight management, which is another crucial factor in controlling hypertension. As excess weight places additional strain on the heart and blood vessels, losing even a small amount of weight through exercise can yield significant improvements in blood pressure readings.

Furthermore, the psychological benefits of regular exercise cannot be overlooked. Physical activity has been linked to reduced stress and anxiety levels, both of which are known contributors to elevated blood pressure. Exercise acts as a natural stress reliever, helping to improve mood and overall mental well-being. This psychological aspect is particularly important for those who may experience hypertension related to stress, as it provides a dual benefit of improving both mental and physical health.

For older adults, incorporating regular exercise into their daily routine can be especially beneficial for blood pressure management. As people age, they may become more sedentary, leading to a decline in cardiovascular health. However, even in older populations, moderate-intensity exercises such as walking, swimming, or cycling can effectively lower blood pressure and promote overall health. It is essential for older adults to consult healthcare providers to tailor an exercise programme that suits their individual capabilities and health conditions.

In conclusion, the impact of regular exercise on blood pressure is profound and multi-dimensional. Not only does it improve physical health by enhancing cardiovascular function, but it also significantly contributes to mental well-being by reducing stress. As part of a comprehensive approach to managing hypertension, incorporating regular physical activity can lead to lasting improvements in blood pressure control and overall health, making it a key recommendation for individuals seeking to manage their hypertension effectively.

Developing an Exercise Routine

Developing a consistent exercise routine is a vital step in managing high blood pressure. Regular physical activity not only helps to lower blood pressure but also contributes to overall cardiovascular health. For individuals with hypertension, incorporating exercise into daily life can be a powerful tool in their health management arsenal. Understanding how to create a sustainable exercise routine is crucial for long-term success in controlling blood pressure levels.

When beginning an exercise regimen, it is essential to consider personal fitness levels and any existing health concerns. A gradual approach is recommended, starting with low-impact activities such as walking, swimming, or cycling. These types of exercises can be easily integrated into daily life and are less likely to cause strain. Setting achievable goals can help maintain motivation and create a sense of accomplishment, which is beneficial for psychological well-being and stress management.

In addition to aerobic activities, strength training should be included in an exercise routine. Research indicates that incorporating resistance exercises at least two days a week can further enhance blood pressure control. It is advisable to consult with a healthcare professional or a certified trainer to ensure that the exercises chosen are safe and effective, particularly for older adults or those with existing health conditions.

Consistency is key when developing an exercise routine. Establishing a specific time each day for physical activity can help build a habit. Engaging in group activities or classes can also provide social support, making the experience more enjoyable. Moreover, tracking progress through a journal or app can serve as a motivator and provide insights into how exercise affects blood pressure readings over time.

Lastly, it is important to remember that any exercise routine should be complemented by other lifestyle changes, such as dietary adjustments and stress management techniques. A holistic approach that includes physical activity, healthy eating, and psychological support can significantly improve outcomes for those managing hypertension. By prioritising a well-rounded routine, individuals can take proactive steps towards better health and well-being.

4

Chapter 4: Psychological Factors and Hypertension

The Link Between Mental Health and Blood Pressure

Mental health and blood pressure are intricately linked, with stress and anxiety often contributing to hypertension. When individuals experience high levels of stress, the body reacts by releasing hormones such as adrenaline and cortisol. These hormones temporarily increase heart rate and blood pressure, which, if experienced chronically, can lead to sustained elevations in blood pressure. Understanding this connection is crucial for effectively managing hypertension and promoting overall well-being.

Psychological factors play a significant role in hypertension management. Conditions such as depression and anxiety can exacerbate high blood pressure, creating a vicious cycle. Individuals struggling with mental health issues may find it challenging to adhere to treatment plans, including medication and lifestyle changes. Thus, addressing mental health is essential for effective blood pressure control and should be considered a vital component of hypertension management strategies.

Dietary approaches to managing hypertension can also be influenced by mental health. For instance, individuals experiencing depression may have a diminished interest in preparing healthy meals or engaging in physical activity, both of which are vital for controlling blood pressure. By improving mental health, individuals may be more motivated to make positive dietary changes, such as adopting a low-sodium diet or incorporating more fruits and vegetables into their meals.

Physical activity is another pivotal aspect of managing both mental health and blood pressure. Regular exercise has been shown to reduce symptoms of anxiety and depression while simultaneously lowering blood pressure levels. Engaging in physical activity releases endorphins, which can enhance mood and contribute to a sense of well-being. Therefore, incorporating regular exercise into daily routines serves as a dual benefit for both mental health and hypertension management.

Lastly, it is important to recognise the impact of sleep on both mental health and blood pressure. Poor sleep quality can lead to increased stress and anxiety, which in turn may elevate blood pressure. Conditions such as sleep apnoea are particularly concerning, as they can disrupt sleep and lead to significant health consequences. Addressing sleep issues through proper management strategies is essential for promoting overall health and effectively controlling hypertension.

Stress Management Techniques

Stress management is essential for everyone, particularly for those managing high blood pressure. Techniques such as deep breathing, meditation, and mindfulness can significantly impact an individual's ability to cope with stress. By incorporating these practices into daily routines, individuals may find a reduction in their overall stress levels, which can contribute to better blood pressure control. Understanding the physiological connection between stress and hypertension is crucial for implementing these techniques effectively.

Physical activity also plays a vital role in stress management. Engaging in regular exercise not only improves cardiovascular health but also helps to alleviate stress. Activities such as walking, swimming, or yoga can provide both physical and mental benefits. Finding an enjoyable form of exercise can motivate individuals to maintain a consistent routine, thereby reducing stress and its potential impact on blood pressure.

Dietary approaches cannot be overlooked when discussing stress management in relation to hypertension. Consuming a balanced diet rich in fruits, vegetables, and whole grains can improve overall health and resilience to stress. Certain foods, such as those high in omega-3 fatty acids, may also help reduce the effects of stress on the body. By combining dietary strategies with stress management techniques, individuals can create a holistic approach to managing their blood pressure.

It is important to consider the psychological factors that contribute to stress and hypertension. Seeking support through counselling or therapy can provide individuals with tools to cope with stress more effectively. Additionally, social connections are vital; engaging with friends and family can offer emotional support and reduce feelings of isolation. Understanding and addressing these psychological aspects can lead to significant improvements in stress levels and blood pressure management.

Lastly, cultivating good sleep hygiene is integral to effective stress management. Poor sleep can exacerbate stress and contribute to high blood pressure, making it essential to prioritise quality sleep. Techniques such as establishing a bedtime routine, minimising screen time before bed, and creating a comfortable sleep environment can promote better sleep quality. By focusing on these various aspects of stress management, individuals can take proactive steps towards maintaining a healthier blood pressure.

The Role of Mindfulness and Relaxation

Mindfulness and relaxation play a crucial role in managing high blood pressure, as they address the psychological factors that significantly influence hypertension. By practising mindfulness, individuals can develop a heightened awareness of their thoughts and feelings, which can help them identify stressors in their lives. This awareness enables them to respond to stress in a more controlled manner, potentially lowering their blood pressure and improving overall health.

Relaxation techniques, such as deep breathing exercises, progressive muscle relaxation, and meditation, have been shown to reduce stress levels and promote a sense of calm. Engaging in these practices regularly can lead to a decrease in the sympathetic nervous system's activity, which is responsible for the body's stress response. As a result, blood vessels can relax, heart rates may stabilise, and blood pressure can be effectively managed over time.

Moreover, the connection between stress and hypertension cannot be overlooked. Chronic stress can lead to unhealthy coping mechanisms, such as overeating, excessive alcohol consumption, or smoking, which all contribute to increased blood pressure. By incorporating mindfulness and relaxation into daily routines, individuals can cultivate healthier habits and reduce the likelihood of these detrimental behaviours, leading to better management of their hypertension.

In addition to the psychological benefits, mindfulness and relaxation techniques can also enhance the effectiveness of dietary and physical activity approaches to managing high blood pressure. When individuals are less stressed, they are more likely to make healthier food choices and maintain a consistent exercise routine. This holistic approach not only aids in controlling blood pressure but also fosters an overall sense of well-being and improves quality of life.

Ultimately, integrating mindfulness and relaxation into the daily lives of those managing high blood pressure can be transformative. By addressing both the mental and physical aspects of hypertension, individuals can take proactive steps towards better health. This comprehensive approach not only empowers individuals to take control of their condition but also encourages a supportive environment where stress management becomes a priority, leading to long-term success in hypertension management.

Seeking Professional Help for Psychological Well-being

The pursuit of psychological well-being is paramount for managing high blood pressure effectively. Individuals often overlook the significant impact that mental health can have on physical health. Stress, anxiety, and depression are all psychological factors that can exacerbate hypertension. Seeking professional help, such as consulting with psychologists or counsellors, can provide individuals with the tools they need to cope with these challenges. By addressing psychological concerns, patients can improve not only their mental health but also their overall cardiovascular health.

Therapeutic interventions can include cognitive behavioural therapy, mindfulness practices, and stress management techniques, all of which have been shown to lower blood pressure. These methods equip individuals with strategies to handle stress more effectively, thereby potentially reducing the need for medication. Professionals can also assist in tailoring dietary and exercise plans that complement mental health treatment, creating a holistic approach to hypertension management. Such integrated care is essential for achieving long-term health benefits.

In addition to therapy, support groups can provide a valuable resource for individuals dealing with high blood pressure. Sharing experiences with others facing similar challenges can foster a sense of community and reduce feelings of isolation. These groups often encourage accountability, motivating members to adhere to healthier lifestyles, which is beneficial for managing hypertension. The emotional support received can be instrumental in reinforcing the importance of maintaining both psychological and physical well-being.

Moreover, recognising when to seek help is crucial. Signs such as persistent sadness, overwhelming stress, or difficulty in coping with daily tasks should prompt individuals to consider professional support. Early intervention can prevent worsening mental health conditions that might lead to increased blood pressure levels. It is essential for individuals to understand that asking for help is a strength, and it plays a vital role in their journey towards better health.

In conclusion, prioritising psychological well-being is not merely an adjunct to managing high blood pressure but a fundamental aspect of effective treatment. By integrating mental health care into hypertension management, individuals can experience improved outcomes. This multifaceted approach ultimately leads to a healthier, more balanced life, where both mind and body are in harmony, significantly reducing the risks associated with high blood pressure.

5

Chapter 5: Hypertension in Older Adults: Risks and Management

Age-Related Changes and Blood Pressure

As individuals age, their bodies undergo various physiological changes, including alterations in the cardiovascular system. One significant change is the stiffening of blood vessels, which can lead to an increase in blood pressure. This process is often exacerbated by the accumulation of plaque in the arteries, a condition known as atherosclerosis. Consequently, older adults are at a higher risk of developing hypertension, making it crucial for them to monitor their blood pressure regularly and engage in preventive measures.

Additionally, age-related changes in the body's hormonal regulation can also affect blood pressure levels. For example, the renin-angiotensin-aldosterone system, which plays a vital role in regulating blood pressure, may become less efficient in older adults. This inefficiency can lead to higher blood pressure readings, further complicating the management of hypertension. Therefore, understanding these changes is essential for both patients and healthcare providers when developing effective treatment strategies.

Lifestyle factors, such as diet and physical activity, also influence blood pressure in older adults. A balanced diet rich in fruits, vegetables, whole grains, and low in sodium can help mitigate age-related increases in blood pressure. Moreover, regular physical activity is crucial as it can improve vascular health and enhance the body's ability to regulate blood pressure. Encouraging older adults to adopt these healthy behaviours is a key component in managing hypertension.

Psychological factors, including stress and anxiety, can have a profound impact on blood pressure, particularly in older individuals. The stress response can trigger the release of hormones that temporarily elevate blood pressure. Therefore, incorporating stress management techniques, such as mindfulness and relaxation exercises, can be beneficial in maintaining healthy blood pressure levels among the elderly.

Finally, the use of medications for managing hypertension in older adults must be approached with caution. Many antihypertensive drugs can have side effects that may be more pronounced in this age group. It is essential for healthcare providers to assess the individual needs of older patients and tailor treatment plans accordingly. Regular monitoring of blood pressure, alongside lifestyle modifications and psychological support, can significantly enhance the quality of life for older adults dealing with hypertension.

Common Comorbidities in Older Adults

As individuals age, the prevalence of comorbidities increases, particularly in relation to hypertension. Common conditions that often coexist with high blood pressure include diabetes, cardiovascular diseases, and kidney disorders. The interplay between these health issues can complicate the management of hypertension, necessitating a comprehensive approach that addresses all underlying conditions. Understanding these comorbidities is crucial for effective treatment and improving patient outcomes.

Diabetes is one of the most frequently encountered comorbidities in older adults with hypertension. The relationship between high blood pressure and diabetes is particularly concerning, as both conditions significantly elevate the risk of cardiovascular events. Managing blood glucose levels and blood pressure simultaneously can be challenging, requiring careful monitoring and adjustments in medication and lifestyle to achieve optimal control.

Cardiovascular diseases, including heart disease and stroke, are also prevalent among older individuals with hypertension. The combination of these conditions often leads to a vicious cycle, where hypertension exacerbates cardiovascular issues while existing heart conditions can further elevate blood pressure. Preventative measures, such as a heart-healthy diet and regular physical activity, are essential in mitigating these risks and promoting overall cardiovascular health.

Kidney disorders, particularly chronic kidney disease, frequently accompany hypertension in the elderly. The kidneys play a vital role in regulating blood pressure, and when compromised, they can contribute to further elevation of blood pressure levels. Consequently, managing kidney health is an integral part of hypertension treatment, which may involve dietary modifications and medication adjustments to ensure both blood pressure and kidney function remain stable.

Lastly, psychological factors such as depression and anxiety are common in older adults with hypertension, often complicating treatment protocols. Stress management and psychological support should be integral components of a comprehensive hypertension management plan. By addressing the psychological aspects alongside physical health, healthcare providers can better support older adults in achieving better control of their blood pressure and overall well-being.

Strategies for Effective Management

Effective management of high blood pressure requires a multifaceted approach that includes lifestyle modifications, medical interventions, and ongoing monitoring. Individuals should first focus on dietary changes, such as adopting a heart-healthy diet rich in fruits, vegetables, whole grains, and low-fat dairy. Reducing sodium intake and limiting processed foods can significantly lower blood pressure levels. These dietary approaches not only help in managing hypertension but also contribute to overall cardiovascular health.

Incorporating regular physical activity is another critical strategy in the management of hypertension. Engaging in at least 150 minutes of moderate-intensity aerobic exercise each week can help lower blood pressure and improve heart function. Activities such as brisk walking, cycling, and swimming not only reduce stress but also enhance mood and promote weight loss, further aiding in blood pressure control. It is essential to find enjoyable activities to ensure consistency and long-term commitment to an active lifestyle.

Psychological factors, including stress and anxiety, play a significant role in hypertension. Developing effective stress management techniques, such as mindfulness, meditation, and deep-breathing exercises, can help mitigate these effects. Additionally, seeking support from mental health professionals can provide valuable tools for coping with stress, ultimately leading to improved blood pressure management. Understanding the connection between emotional well-being and physical health is vital for those managing hypertension.

For older adults, tailored management strategies are crucial due to the increased risks associated with hypertension in this demographic. Regular monitoring of blood pressure, along with a focus on medication adherence, is essential for effective control. Healthcare providers should work closely with older patients to customise treatment plans that consider their unique health needs, potential side effects of medications, and the impact of comorbidities on blood pressure management.

Lastly, understanding the role of sleep in blood pressure regulation cannot be overlooked. Conditions such as sleep apnoea can exacerbate hypertension, making it imperative to address sleep quality and quantity. Individuals should be encouraged to establish healthy sleep habits and seek medical evaluation for sleep disorders if necessary. Overall, a comprehensive and proactive approach to managing hypertension through lifestyle changes, psychological support, and medical care is essential for long-term health and well-being.

Importance of Regular Monitoring

Regular monitoring of blood pressure is essential for everyone, particularly for those at risk of hypertension. High blood pressure often presents no symptoms, making it crucial to check levels regularly to detect any abnormalities early. By tracking blood pressure consistently, individuals can gain insights into their cardiovascular health and take proactive steps to manage it effectively. Understanding one's blood pressure readings empowers individuals to make informed lifestyle changes and seek medical advice when necessary.

In the context of dietary approaches to managing hypertension, regular monitoring plays a pivotal role. Individuals can observe how specific dietary changes affect their blood pressure. For instance, reducing salt intake or increasing potassium-rich foods can lead to significant improvements. By keeping a close eye on blood pressure readings, one can assess the effectiveness of these dietary adjustments, allowing for a more tailored approach to managing hypertension.

Physical activity is another critical factor in controlling blood pressure, and monitoring helps to establish a connection between exercise and blood pressure levels. By recording blood pressure before and after physical activity, individuals can identify the positive impact of regular exercise on their blood pressure. This knowledge can motivate individuals to maintain an active lifestyle, contributing to long-term cardiovascular health.

Psychological factors and stress management are also intertwined with blood pressure regulation. Regular monitoring can help individuals recognise how stress levels affect their blood pressure. This awareness can encourage the adoption of stress-reduction techniques such as meditation or mindfulness, which may lead to better blood pressure control. Moreover, monitoring can serve as a feedback mechanism, reinforcing the importance of psychological well-being in managing hypertension.

For older adults, the risks associated with hypertension are particularly pronounced, making regular monitoring even more vital. As the body ages, blood vessels may become stiffer, leading to higher blood pressure readings.

Regular checks can help in identifying trends and make necessary adjustments in treatment or lifestyle. This proactive approach can enhance quality of life and reduce the risk of complications associated with high blood pressure, underscoring the importance of consistent monitoring in the management of hypertension.

6

Chapter 6: Understanding the Impact of Stress on Blood Pressure

The Physiology of Stress Response

The physiology of stress response is a complex interplay of biological mechanisms that are activated when an individual perceives a threat. This response is primarily mediated by the autonomic nervous system, which is responsible for involuntary bodily functions. When faced with stress, the hypothalamus signals the adrenal glands to release hormones such as adrenaline and cortisol. These hormones prepare the body to respond to the challenge, resulting in increased heart rate, elevated blood pressure, and heightened alertness. Understanding this response is crucial for recognising its impact on overall health, particularly concerning hypertension.

Chronic stress can lead to sustained high levels of these hormones, which may contribute to the development of hypertension. The constant activation of the stress response can result in physiological changes such as increased vascular resistance and alterations in heart function. Over time, these changes can damage blood vessels and lead to the stiffening of arteries, which are significant risk factors for hypertension. Therefore, managing stress is essential not only for mental well-being but also for maintaining healthy blood pressure levels.

Moreover, psychological factors play a pivotal role in stress response and its effects on blood pressure. Individuals with anxiety or depression may experience heightened stress responses, which can exacerbate hypertension. This interconnection highlights the importance of addressing mental health in the management of high blood pressure. Strategies such as cognitive-behavioural therapy, mindfulness, and relaxation techniques can be beneficial in mitigating stress and its physiological effects.

Physical activity also emerges as a critical factor in managing stress response. Regular exercise can help lower levels of stress hormones and promote the release of endorphins, which enhance mood and promote relaxation. Engaging in physical activity not only counteracts the negative effects of stress but also contributes to better cardiovascular health, making it an essential component in the management of hypertension. Incorporating regular exercise into daily routines can therefore serve as a preventive measure against the adverse effects of stress on blood pressure.

In conclusion, understanding the physiology of stress response is vital for grasping its implications for hypertension. The body's reaction to stress involves a cascade of hormonal changes that can adversely affect cardiovascular health. By managing stress through psychological interventions and physical activity, individuals can better control their blood pressure and reduce the risk of hypertension-related complications. This holistic approach ensures that both mental and physical health are addressed, leading to improved overall well-being.

Identifying Sources of Stress

Stress is an omnipresent factor in modern life, influencing various aspects of health, including blood pressure. Identifying sources of stress is essential for managing hypertension effectively. Common stressors can range from work-related pressures to personal relationships and financial concerns. By recognising these triggers, individuals can take proactive steps to mitigate their impact on overall health and wellbeing.

One of the primary sources of stress for many people is their work environment. High demands, tight deadlines, and interpersonal conflicts can contribute to elevated stress levels, leading to increased blood pressure. It is crucial for individuals to assess their work-life balance and identify specific stressors that may be contributing to their hypertension. Implementing stress management techniques in the workplace can be beneficial in reducing these pressures.

Personal relationships also play a significant role in stress levels. Whether it is conflicts with family members, friends, or partners, interpersonal issues can create emotional turmoil that affects both mental and physical health. Understanding how these relationships impact one's stress levels can lead to healthier communication strategies and conflict resolution methods, ultimately aiding in the management of blood pressure.

Financial concerns are another prevalent source of stress that can have a detrimental effect on health. Worries about income, debt, and financial stability can lead to chronic stress, which is closely linked to hypertension. By developing a financial plan and seeking support, individuals can alleviate some of this stress, contributing to better blood pressure control.

Lastly, lifestyle factors such as poor sleep patterns, lack of physical activity, and unhealthy dietary choices can exacerbate stress and, consequently, hypertension. Recognising these lifestyle-related stressors is vital for developing a comprehensive approach to managing blood pressure. Encouraging healthy habits and self-care practices can significantly reduce stress levels, leading to improved overall health and wellbeing.

Long-term Effects of Chronic Stress

Chronic stress is a pervasive issue that can have profound long-term effects on both mental and physical health. When individuals are exposed to continuous stressors, their bodies remain in a heightened state of alertness, leading to an array of physiological responses. These responses can result in increased heart rates, elevated blood pressure, and a surge in stress hormones, which are all detrimental to overall health. Over time, this constant state of stress can contribute to the development of hypertension, a condition that affects millions of individuals worldwide.

The relationship between chronic stress and hypertension is particularly concerning for older adults, who may already be at a higher risk for developing high blood pressure due to age-related factors. As stress continues to impact their health, older adults may find themselves facing compounded risks, including heart disease and stroke. Understanding the role that stress plays in blood pressure regulation is crucial for managing hypertension effectively in this demographic. Furthermore, it highlights the need for comprehensive strategies that address both psychological and physiological aspects of health.

Dietary approaches to managing hypertension can also be influenced by stress levels. Many individuals under chronic stress may resort to unhealthy eating habits, such as consuming high-sugar or high-sodium foods, which can further exacerbate blood pressure issues. Implementing a balanced diet rich in fruits, vegetables, and whole grains can help mitigate these effects and promote better blood pressure control. This dietary shift not only supports physical health but can also serve as a coping mechanism to reduce stress levels.

Physical activity is another critical element in managing the effects of chronic stress on blood pressure. Regular exercise has been shown to lower stress hormones, improve mood, and enhance overall cardiovascular health. For those dealing with chronic stress, engaging in physical activities such as walking, swimming, or yoga can provide significant relief and contribute to better blood pressure management. Thus, incorporating exercise into daily routines is essential for those looking to combat the long-term effects of stress on their health.

Lastly, it is important to recognise the psychological factors that interplay with hypertension. Chronic stress not only affects physical health but also has a significant impact on mental well-being. Addressing the psychological aspects of stress through techniques such as mindfulness, therapy, and relaxation exercises can lead to more effective hypertension management. By adopting a holistic approach that encompasses diet, exercise, and mental health, individuals can better navigate the complexities of chronic stress and its long-term effects on blood pressure.

Stress Reduction Techniques

Stress is a significant factor that can contribute to high blood pressure, and understanding how to manage it effectively is crucial for maintaining cardiovascular health. Various stress reduction techniques can help individuals lower their blood pressure and improve overall well-being. These techniques range from mindfulness practices to physical activities that promote relaxation, making them accessible to everyone regardless of their lifestyle or background.

One of the most effective methods for reducing stress is mindfulness meditation. This practice encourages individuals to focus on the present moment and become aware of their thoughts and feelings without judgment. Regular mindfulness meditation can decrease stress hormones and promote a sense of calm, which can be beneficial for those managing hypertension. It can easily be incorporated into daily routines, even for just a few minutes at a time.

Physical activity is another vital component of stress reduction. Engaging in regular exercise not only helps to lower blood pressure but also releases endorphins, the body's natural mood lifters. Activities such as walking, swimming, or yoga can provide both physical and mental benefits. The combination of movement and the focus required during these activities can serve as a powerful distraction from stressors, fostering a more relaxed state of mind.

In addition to mindfulness and physical activity, social support plays a key role in stress management. Connecting with friends and family can provide emotional support and help alleviate feelings of isolation that may arise from stress. Group activities or support groups focused on health and wellness can also encourage individuals to share their experiences and coping strategies, creating a sense of community that is essential for mental health.

Finally, prioritising sleep is crucial for effective stress management. Poor sleep can exacerbate stress and negatively impact blood pressure levels. Establishing a regular sleep schedule, creating a restful environment, and practising good sleep hygiene can significantly improve sleep quality. This, in turn, can lead to better stress management and lower blood pressure, contributing to overall health and well-being.

7

Chapter 7: Medications for Hypertension: Types and Side Effects and How They Work

Overview of Antihypertensive Medications

Antihypertensive medications play a crucial role in managing high blood pressure, a condition that affects millions worldwide. These medications are designed to lower blood pressure and reduce the risk of complications such as heart attacks and strokes. There are various classes of antihypertensive drugs, each working through different mechanisms to achieve optimal blood pressure control. Understanding the different types of medications available is essential for patients and healthcare providers alike.

The primary classes of antihypertensive medications include diuretics, ACE inhibitors, angiotensin II receptor blockers (ARBs), calcium channel blockers, and beta-blockers. Diuretics help eliminate excess fluid and sodium from the body, which can lower blood pressure. ACE inhibitors and ARBs work by relaxing blood vessels, making it easier for the heart to pump blood. Calcium channel blockers reduce the heart's workload by preventing calcium from entering the cells of the heart and blood vessels. Beta-blockers decrease heart rate and the heart's output of blood.

While these medications are effective, they are not without potential side effects. Common side effects may include dizziness, fatigue, and gastrointestinal issues. Some individuals may experience more severe reactions, such as allergic responses or electrolyte imbalances. It is essential for patients to discuss any side effects with their healthcare provider to determine the best course of action. Additionally, lifestyle changes should complement medication use for optimal management of hypertension.

Monitoring blood pressure regularly is vital for anyone on antihypertensive medication. Home devices can offer a convenient way to keep track of blood pressure readings, but they should not replace clinical measurements. Regular check-ups with a healthcare provider ensure that the treatment plan is effective and adjusted as necessary. Proper management can lead to improved health outcomes and a better quality of life for individuals with hypertension.

In conclusion, antihypertensive medications are a cornerstone in the treatment of high blood pressure. With various options available, patients can work with their healthcare providers to find the most suitable medication based on their specific needs and health conditions. Understanding the mechanisms, potential side effects, and the importance of regular monitoring can empower patients to take charge of their health and manage their hypertension effectively.

Common Classes of Medications

High blood pressure, or hypertension, can often be managed effectively with a variety of medications. Understanding the common classes of medications available is crucial for anyone seeking to control their blood pressure. These medications work in different ways to lower blood pressure, and each class has its own mechanism of action, benefits, and potential side effects. Patients should be aware of these options, as they play a significant role in the overall management of hypertension and can influence lifestyle choices and dietary approaches.

One of the most commonly prescribed classes of medications for hypertension is diuretics. These drugs help the body eliminate excess sodium and water through urine, which can reduce blood volume and, consequently, blood pressure. By lowering the volume of blood circulating in the body, diuretics can effectively decrease the strain on the heart and blood vessels. However, while they are generally well-tolerated, patients may experience side effects such as dehydration and electrolyte imbalances, which should be monitored closely.

Another important class of medications is ACE inhibitors. These drugs work by blocking the action of angiotensin-converting enzyme, which is responsible for the production of a hormone that narrows blood vessels. By preventing this hormone from forming, ACE inhibitors promote relaxation of the blood vessels, leading to lower blood pressure. Though these medications are often effective, they can cause side effects, including a persistent cough and elevated potassium levels, necessitating regular monitoring.

Calcium channel blockers also play a significant role in hypertension management. They function by blocking calcium from entering the cells of the heart and blood vessels, leading to a decrease in heart rate and dilation of the blood vessels. This results in reduced blood pressure and improved blood flow. While generally effective, some individuals may experience side effects such as swelling of the ankles and flushing, which may warrant a discussion with their healthcare provider for potential adjustments in dosage or medication type.

Lastly, beta-blockers are another class of medication often used to treat high blood pressure. These drugs reduce the heart rate and the force of the heart's contractions, ultimately decreasing the amount of blood pumped through the blood vessels. While effective for many, beta-blockers can cause fatigue and a decrease in exercise tolerance, which is a crucial consideration for individuals focusing on physical activity as part of their hypertension management plan. Overall, understanding the various classes of medications available allows patients to engage in informed discussions with their healthcare providers, aligning their treatment plans with their lifestyle and health goals.

ACE Inhibitors & ARBs: relax vessels, block RAAS

ACE inhibitors and angiotensin receptor blockers (ARBs) are pivotal in managing hypertension, particularly due to their ability to relax blood vessels. These medications target the renin-angiotensin-aldosterone system (RAAS), a hormone system that regulates blood pressure and fluid balance. By inhibiting the conversion of angiotensin I to angiotensin II, ACE inhibitors prevent blood vessels from narrowing, which can significantly lower blood pressure levels. Similarly, ARBs block the action of angiotensin II directly at its receptor sites, allowing blood vessels to remain dilated and reducing the strain on the heart.

The role of these medications in hypertension management cannot be overstated. They not only help in lowering blood pressure but also provide protective benefits for the heart and kidneys. By alleviating the workload on the cardiovascular system, individuals taking ACE inhibitors or ARBs may experience a reduced risk of developing complications associated with high blood pressure, such as heart attacks, strokes, and kidney disease. This dual action makes them a preferred choice for many healthcare providers.

In addition to their pharmacological effects, lifestyle modifications can further enhance the efficacy of these medications. Diet plays a crucial role in managing blood pressure, with a focus on reducing sodium intake while increasing potassium-rich foods. Regular physical activity is also essential, as it helps to maintain a healthy weight and improves overall cardiovascular health. Implementing these dietary and activity changes alongside ACE inhibitors or ARBs can lead to better control of hypertension.

Psychological factors, such as stress and anxiety, can also impact blood pressure levels. It is vital for patients to engage in stress-reducing techniques, such as mindfulness and relaxation exercises, to complement their medical treatment. Additionally, understanding the connection between sleep apnoea and hypertension highlights the need for a comprehensive approach to managing this condition. Addressing all these factors not only aids in controlling blood pressure but also improves the quality of life for individuals.

Monitoring blood pressure is crucial for those prescribed ACE inhibitors or ARBs. Patients should regularly check their blood pressure at home and maintain communication with their healthcare providers to adjust treatment as necessary. Awareness of the potential side effects of these medications, such as dizziness or changes in kidney function, is also important. By staying informed and proactive in managing their health, individuals can effectively navigate the complexities of hypertension treatment and improve their long-term outcomes.

Calcium Channel Blockers - reduce vascular resistance

Calcium channel blockers (CCBs) are a class of medications that play a significant role in managing high blood pressure by reducing vascular resistance. They work by inhibiting the influx of calcium ions into the smooth muscle cells of the blood vessels, which causes relaxation and dilation. This dilation helps to lower the overall resistance that blood encounters as it flows through the circulatory system, ultimately leading to decreased blood pressure levels. Understanding how CCBs function is crucial for those looking to manage hypertension effectively.

One of the key benefits of calcium channel blockers is their ability to selectively target the vascular smooth muscle without significantly affecting the heart rate. This makes them particularly useful for patients who may be at risk for heart-related side effects associated with other antihypertensive medications. By relaxing the blood vessels, CCBs can improve blood flow and reduce the workload on the heart, making them an important option for diverse patient populations, including older adults.

In addition to their direct effects on blood pressure, CCBs may also offer ancillary benefits for patients with coexisting conditions, such as angina or certain types of arrhythmias. Their ability to improve blood flow can alleviate symptoms associated with these conditions, thus providing a dual benefit for individuals managing multiple health issues. When combined with dietary approaches and lifestyle modifications, the effectiveness of CCBs can be enhanced significantly.

It is essential for patients to be aware of the possible side effects associated with calcium channel blockers, which may include swelling in the legs, dizziness, or flushing. These side effects can vary among individuals, and it is advisable to discuss any concerns with a healthcare provider to ensure that the chosen medication aligns with personal health needs and lifestyle. Monitoring blood pressure regularly can also help in assessing the effectiveness of the treatment plan.

Ultimately, reducing vascular resistance through the use of calcium channel blockers is a valuable strategy in the comprehensive management of hypertension. By working in tandem with lifestyle changes and dietary adjustments, these medications can help individuals achieve and maintain healthy blood pressure levels. Understanding the role of CCBs not only empowers patients but also enhances their ability to take an active part in their health management journey.

Diuretics: reduce blood volume

Diuretics, commonly referred to as "water pills," play a significant role in managing high blood pressure by reducing blood volume. These medications encourage the kidneys to excrete more sodium and water, which subsequently lowers the fluid in the bloodstream. As a result, the heart does not have to work as hard to pump blood, leading to a reduction in blood pressure. Understanding how diuretics function is essential for anyone looking to manage hypertension effectively, especially in conjunction with lifestyle changes such as diet and exercise.

The primary types of diuretics include thiazide, loop, and potassium-sparing diuretics, each with unique mechanisms and indications. Thiazide diuretics are often the first line of treatment for hypertension, known for their effectiveness in lowering blood pressure while also promoting heart health. Loop diuretics, on the other hand, are typically used in patients with heart failure or fluid retention, while potassium-sparing diuretics help maintain potassium levels, which can be crucial for overall health. Understanding these differences can aid in selecting the appropriate diuretic for individual needs.

While diuretics are beneficial, they may also come with side effects that patients should be aware of. Common side effects include dehydration, electrolyte imbalances, and increased urination, which can lead to discomfort and inconvenience. Patients should monitor their hydration levels and report any unusual symptoms to their healthcare provider. Maintaining open communication with a healthcare professional can help manage these side effects effectively while still reaping the benefits of diuretic therapy.

In addition to medication, lifestyle modifications are essential in managing hypertension. A balanced diet rich in fruits, vegetables, and low in sodium can enhance the efficacy of diuretics. Regular physical activity not only supports weight management but also improves cardiovascular health, further aiding in blood pressure control. Psychological factors, including stress management and adequate sleep, also play a critical role in maintaining healthy blood pressure levels, underscoring the multifaceted approach required for effective hypertension management.

For older adults, diuretics can be particularly beneficial, yet they must be used cautiously due to the increased risk of dehydration and falls. Regular monitoring of blood pressure and kidney function is vital in this population, as age-related changes can affect how medications are processed in the body. By combining pharmacological treatments like diuretics with lifestyle adjustments and regular medical supervision, individuals can achieve better control over their hypertension and enhance their overall quality of life.

Beta Blockers: slow heart rate and reduce cardiac output

Beta blockers are a class of medications commonly prescribed to manage high blood pressure. They work by blocking the effects of adrenaline on the heart, leading to a slower heart rate and reduced cardiac output. This mechanism is particularly beneficial for individuals who experience elevated blood pressure due to stress or anxiety, as it helps to calm the heart and reduce the overall workload on the cardiovascular system.

By lowering the heart rate, beta blockers can effectively decrease the amount of blood pumped through the arteries with each heartbeat. This reduction in cardiac output not only aids in controlling hypertension but also contributes to improved heart function in patients with certain heart conditions. For those with hypertension, particularly older adults, the use of beta blockers can offer a significant advantage in managing blood pressure levels and minimising the risks associated with uncontrolled hypertension.

Moreover, beta blockers are often part of a comprehensive approach to hypertension management that includes dietary changes and increased physical activity. Adopting a heart-healthy diet can complement the effects of beta blockers, while regular physical activity can enhance cardiovascular health. This holistic approach is crucial in addressing not just the symptoms of hypertension but also its underlying causes.

It is important for patients to understand the potential side effects of beta blockers, which can include fatigue, cold extremities, and sometimes depression. Monitoring blood pressure regularly is essential to evaluate the effectiveness of the medication and to make any necessary adjustments. This ongoing assessment can aid in determining whether the benefits of beta blockers outweigh any adverse effects experienced by the patient.

In summary, beta blockers play a significant role in the management of hypertension by slowing the heart rate and reducing cardiac output. These medications can be particularly effective for individuals who have additional risk factors like stress and anxiety. As part of a broader strategy for managing high blood pressure, they contribute to improved health outcomes and a better quality of life for those affected by this condition.

Alpha Blockers: Centrally Acting Agents

Alpha blockers are a class of medications that primarily work by blocking alpha-adrenergic receptors in the central nervous system. This action leads to a decrease in peripheral vascular resistance, which can help lower blood pressure. By relaxing the blood vessels, alpha blockers facilitate smoother blood flow, making them a valuable option in the management of hypertension. Although they are not the first line of treatment, they can be particularly beneficial for certain patient populations, especially those with comorbid conditions.

These medications can be particularly effective for individuals who experience hypertension associated with conditions such as benign prostatic hyperplasia (BPH). Alpha blockers can alleviate urinary symptoms while simultaneously managing blood pressure, creating a dual benefit for patients. However, it is essential for healthcare providers to consider the overall health profile of patients before prescribing these agents, as they may not be suitable for everyone.

Patients using alpha blockers may experience side effects, including dizziness, fatigue, and headaches. These side effects occur due to the medication's influence on blood pressure regulation and vascular tone. It is crucial for patients to communicate any adverse effects with their healthcare providers, who can then adjust dosages or consider alternative therapies. Monitoring is especially important in older adults, who may be more susceptible to these side effects due to age-related physiological changes.

In addition to pharmacological treatment, lifestyle modifications play a significant role in managing hypertension. Dietary approaches, such as reducing sodium intake and increasing potassium-rich foods, can complement the effects of alpha blockers. Furthermore, engaging in regular physical activity can enhance cardiovascular health and further aid in blood pressure control. Stress management techniques, including mindfulness and relaxation exercises, can also be beneficial for individuals dealing with hypertension.

Ultimately, while alpha blockers are effective in treating hypertension, they should be part of a comprehensive approach that includes both medication and lifestyle changes. Regular monitoring of blood pressure, whether through home devices or clinical measurements, is essential to assess the efficacy of the treatment plan. By understanding the role of alpha blockers and integrating them into a broader strategy, patients can achieve better control over their blood pressure and overall health.

Direct Vasodilators: for resistant cases

Direct vasodilators represent a crucial class of medications used in managing resistant hypertension, which is a condition where blood pressure remains high despite treatment with multiple antihypertensive agents. These medications work by directly relaxing the smooth muscles within blood vessel walls, leading to a reduction in vascular resistance and, consequently, a decrease in blood pressure. This mechanism is particularly beneficial for patients who have not responded adequately to other forms of treatment, providing an alternative approach to achieving better blood pressure control.

Commonly used direct vasodilators include hydralazine and minoxidil, each with its specific indications and side effects. For instance, hydralazine is often employed in cases of hypertension during pregnancy, while minoxidil is generally reserved for severe cases due to its potent effects. Both medications require careful monitoring due to potential side effects, such as reflex tachycardia and fluid retention, necessitating the concurrent use of diuretics and beta-blockers to mitigate these risks.

The role of direct vasodilators extends beyond mere blood pressure reduction; they also play a part in improving overall cardiovascular health. By effectively lowering blood pressure, these medications can help reduce the strain on the heart and other organs, decreasing the risk of complications such as heart failure, stroke, and kidney damage. This is particularly important for older adults, who are often more susceptible to the adverse effects of hypertension due to age-related changes in vascular structure and function.

When considering the use of direct vasodilators, healthcare providers must assess the individual patient's context, including lifestyle factors such as diet and physical activity. For example, integrating dietary approaches, like the DASH diet, alongside pharmacological treatment can enhance blood pressure management. Additionally, understanding the psychological factors that contribute to hypertension can also inform a more comprehensive treatment strategy, as stress management techniques may complement the effects of medications.

In conclusion, while direct vasodilators are an essential tool in the management of resistant hypertension, they are most effective when used as part of a holistic approach to treatment. This includes regular monitoring of blood pressure, lifestyle modifications, and addressing any underlying psychological factors. By adopting a comprehensive strategy, patients can achieve better control of their blood pressure, thereby reducing their risk of serious health complications associated with hypertension.

Combination Therapy: Why It's Often Needed

Combination therapy for hypertension is often necessary due to the complex nature of blood pressure regulation in the body. High blood pressure, or hypertension, is influenced by various factors including genetics, diet, and lifestyle. As individuals respond differently to medications, relying on a single treatment may not adequately control blood pressure levels for everyone. Therefore, utilising a combination of therapies can enhance effectiveness and cater to individual needs, making it a critical component in hypertension management.

The role of dietary approaches and physical activity cannot be underestimated when discussing combination therapy. A balanced diet rich in fruits, vegetables, and whole grains, alongside regular physical exercise, can significantly impact blood pressure control. These lifestyle changes often complement medication, creating a synergistic effect that can lead to improved outcomes. Furthermore, integrating psychological factors into treatment, such as stress management and mental health support, can enhance the overall effectiveness of combination therapy.

In older adults, the need for combination therapy becomes even more pronounced. As people age, their bodies may react differently to medications, and they are often managing multiple health conditions simultaneously. Combination therapy allows healthcare providers to tailor treatments that address both hypertension and any coexisting medical issues, reducing the risk of side effects and improving patient compliance. This holistic approach is vital in ensuring effective management of blood pressure in older populations.

Monitoring and adjusting combination therapy is also essential. Regular blood pressure measurements, whether at home or in clinical settings, help determine the effectiveness of the current regimen and guide necessary adjustments. Patients should be encouraged to engage in this process, thereby fostering a proactive approach to their health management. This continuous monitoring ensures that treatment remains effective over time, accommodating any changes in the patient's health status or lifestyle.

In summary, combination therapy is often necessary in managing hypertension due to the multifaceted nature of the condition. By integrating dietary changes, physical activity, psychological support, and careful monitoring, healthcare providers can create a comprehensive treatment plan that addresses the unique needs of each individual. This approach not only optimises blood pressure control but also enhances the overall quality of life for patients battling hypertension.

Side Effects and Considerations

High blood pressure, or hypertension, can come with a range of side effects and considerations that are crucial for individuals to understand. One of the most common side effects associated with hypertension is the increased risk of cardiovascular diseases. These can manifest as heart attacks or strokes, which often occur silently until it is too late. Therefore, it is essential to monitor blood pressure regularly and remain aware of the symptoms that may indicate complications arising from prolonged high blood pressure.

In addition to cardiovascular concerns, hypertension can also affect other bodily systems. For instance, chronic high blood pressure can lead to kidney damage, resulting in reduced kidney function or even kidney failure over time. This connection underscores the importance of managing blood pressure not just for heart health but for overall bodily function. Patients should engage in discussions with healthcare providers about potential renal implications and appropriate monitoring strategies.

Dietary approaches play a significant role in managing hypertension, and individuals should be aware of the side effects of certain dietary choices. High sodium intake, for example, can exacerbate high blood pressure, while a diet rich in fruits, vegetables, and whole grains can help in lowering it. Educating oneself on how dietary habits influence blood pressure can empower individuals to make informed choices that contribute to better health outcomes.

Moreover, psychological factors, such as stress and anxiety, can significantly impact blood pressure levels. Individuals with high stress may experience spikes in blood pressure, leading to a cycle of worsening health. Incorporating stress management techniques, such as mindfulness and regular physical activity, can mitigate these effects and promote a healthier lifestyle overall. Understanding the psychological aspects of hypertension is essential for comprehensive management.

Lastly, certain medications prescribed for hypertension also come with their own set of side effects that patients should consider. These may include dizziness, fatigue, or even more severe reactions in some cases. It is crucial for patients to communicate openly with their healthcare providers about any adverse effects they experience and to discuss potential alternatives if necessary. A well-rounded approach to managing hypertension requires awareness of these medications and their implications on overall health.

Adherence to Medication Regimen

Adherence to a prescribed medication regimen is crucial for individuals managing high blood pressure. Many patients may underestimate the importance of consistently taking their medications, leading to fluctuations in blood pressure levels that can have serious health implications. Understanding the role of medication in hypertension management helps patients recognise that maintaining a regular schedule is vital for controlling their condition effectively.

Several factors can influence a patient's adherence to their medication regimen. These may include side effects, the complexity of the dosing schedule, and a lack of understanding about the necessity of the treatment. Educating patients about their medications, including how and when to take them, can significantly improve adherence rates. Additionally, addressing any concerns about side effects can help patients feel more comfortable with their treatment plans.

Support systems play an essential role in encouraging adherence. Family members, friends, and healthcare providers can provide reminders and emotional support to help patients stay on track. Group support sessions can also be beneficial, allowing individuals to share experiences and strategies for overcoming challenges related to their medication regimen. Creating an environment where patients feel supported can lead to better health outcomes.

Monitoring blood pressure regularly is another critical aspect of adherence. Patients who track their blood pressure using home devices can gain immediate feedback on how well their medication is working. This self-monitoring empowers patients to take control of their health and encourages them to remain committed to their prescribed regimen. Regular check-ups with healthcare professionals also reinforce the importance of adherence and provide opportunities to make necessary adjustments.

In conclusion, adherence to a medication regimen is a cornerstone of effective hypertension management. By understanding the importance of their medications, utilising support systems, and monitoring their progress, patients can improve their health outcomes significantly. With the right tools and knowledge, individuals can manage their high blood pressure effectively and lead healthier lives.

8

Chapter 8: Monitoring Blood Pressure: Home Devices vs. Clinical Measurements

Importance of Regular Blood Pressure Monitoring

Regular blood pressure monitoring is essential for everyone, as it serves as a critical tool in the early detection and management of hypertension. Hypertension is often referred to as a silent killer because it can develop without noticeable symptoms. By regularly checking blood pressure, individuals can gain valuable insights into their cardiovascular health and take proactive steps to prevent potential complications.

For those managing hypertension through dietary approaches, understanding blood pressure readings can guide dietary choices. Foods rich in potassium, magnesium, and fibre can help lower blood pressure, while high-sodium foods can exacerbate the condition. Regular monitoring allows individuals to assess how dietary changes impact their blood pressure, reinforcing the importance of a balanced diet in hypertension management.

Physical activity plays a significant role in controlling blood pressure, and monitoring can help track the effectiveness of exercise routines. Engaging in regular physical activity can lead to significant improvements in blood pressure levels. By keeping a record of blood pressure before and after workouts, individuals can identify which activities yield the best results, encouraging consistency and motivation in their fitness journey.

Psychological factors, such as stress and anxiety, can also influence blood pressure levels. Regular monitoring provides feedback on how stress management techniques, like mindfulness or relaxation exercises, affect blood pressure. This awareness can empower individuals to adopt healthier coping mechanisms, ultimately improving both their mental and cardiovascular health.

For older adults, regular blood pressure monitoring is particularly crucial due to the increased risk associated with age. Conditions such as sleep apnoea and hypertension can occur together, complicating management strategies. By keeping track of blood pressure regularly, older adults can work closely with healthcare providers to tailor their treatment plans, ensuring a comprehensive approach to managing both hypertension and related health issues.

Types of Monitoring Devices

Monitoring devices play a crucial role in the management of high blood pressure by providing consistent and accurate readings. These devices come in various types, each designed to cater to different needs and preferences of users. Understanding the available options is essential for individuals aiming to keep their blood pressure within a healthy range, especially those diagnosed with hypertension or at risk of developing it.

The most common type of monitoring device is the sphygmomanometer, which can be manual or digital. Manual devices require a stethoscope and a certain level of skill to operate effectively, while digital monitors offer ease of use with automatic readings. Many people prefer digital monitors for home use due to their convenience and the ability to store multiple readings, which aids in tracking blood pressure over time.

Another popular option is the wrist blood pressure monitor, which is compact and portable, making it suitable for individuals who travel frequently or have limited space. These devices are user-friendly but may be less accurate than upper arm monitors due to variations in wrist size and positioning. It is important to follow the manufacturer's instructions to ensure reliable measurements when using wrist monitors.

For those who require continuous monitoring, ambulatory blood pressure monitors are available. These devices are worn for 24 hours and take readings at regular intervals, providing a comprehensive overview of blood pressure fluctuations throughout daily activities. They are particularly useful for diagnosing conditions like white coat hypertension, where individuals experience elevated readings in clinical settings but normal levels at home.

In recent years, smart technology has entered the realm of blood pressure monitoring, with devices that can connect to smartphones and other digital platforms. These smart monitors not only record blood pressure but also allow users to track their health data over time, set reminders for medication, and share results with healthcare providers. This integration of technology facilitates a proactive approach to managing hypertension, empowering individuals to take control of their health.

How to Accurately Measure Blood Pressure at Home

Measuring blood pressure at home is an essential skill for individuals managing hypertension. It allows for consistent monitoring and helps in understanding how lifestyle changes, dietary adjustments, and medications are affecting overall blood pressure levels. To start, it's crucial to choose an appropriate blood pressure monitor that is validated for accuracy. Automatic digital monitors are recommended for ease of use, especially for those who may struggle with reading traditional sphygmomanometers.

Before taking a measurement, prepare by sitting quietly for a few minutes in a comfortable position with your back supported and feet flat on the floor. Ensure that your arm is at heart level, and the cuff is placed correctly on the upper arm, following the manufacturer's instructions. Consistency is key, so try to measure blood pressure at the same time each day to track changes accurately. Avoid caffeine, exercise, and smoking for at least 30 minutes prior to measurement, as these factors can elevate blood pressure temporarily.

When you are ready to measure, press the start button on the monitor and remain still while it inflates and deflates the cuff. The device will display your systolic and diastolic readings, along with your heart rate. It's advisable to take two or three readings, waiting a minute between each, and record the results. This practice can provide a more accurate representation of your blood pressure, as single readings can be influenced by temporary factors such as stress or anxiety.

Regularly monitoring your blood pressure at home not only empowers you to manage your health but also provides valuable information to share with your healthcare provider. This data can help them adjust medications or recommend lifestyle changes more effectively. Additionally, being aware of your blood pressure patterns can help identify triggers related to dietary choices, physical activity, or psychological stress, which are all important elements in managing hypertension.

Lastly, remember that while home monitoring is beneficial, it does not replace regular check-ups with your healthcare provider. Always discuss your readings with them, especially if you notice significant changes or consistently high readings. Combining home monitoring with professional guidance ensures a comprehensive approach to managing high blood pressure and improving overall health.

Understanding Blood Pressure Readings

Blood pressure readings are crucial in understanding an individual's cardiovascular health. They are typically presented in two numbers: systolic and diastolic pressure. The systolic pressure, the higher of the two, measures the force of blood against artery walls when the heart beats. In contrast, the diastolic pressure gauges this same force when the heart is at rest between beats. Recognising these two components helps in comprehending the overall blood pressure reading and its implications for health.

Understanding what constitutes normal, elevated, and hypertensive readings is essential for everyone. A normal blood pressure reading is generally considered to be around 120/80 mmHg. Elevated readings, which range from 120-129 systolic and less than 80 diastolic, may not require medication but indicate a need for lifestyle changes. Hypertension is classified into stages; Stage 1 is indicated by readings of 130-139 systolic or 80-89 diastolic, while Stage 2 is defined as 140/90 mmHg or higher. Recognising these categories can empower individuals to take proactive steps toward maintaining or improving their health.

Monitoring blood pressure regularly is vital for those at risk of hypertension, including older adults and those with certain health conditions. Home monitoring devices have become increasingly popular, allowing individuals to track their blood pressure conveniently. However, it is crucial to ensure that these devices are accurate and used correctly. Clinical measurements taken by healthcare professionals still play a significant role in diagnosis and management, especially when evaluating the effectiveness of treatments or lifestyle modifications.

Lifestyle factors, such as diet and physical activity, significantly influence blood pressure readings. A diet rich in fruits, vegetables, and low-fat dairy, combined with reduced salt intake, can lead to notable improvements in blood pressure. Moreover, regular physical activity not only aids in weight management but also strengthens the heart and improves its efficiency in pumping blood. Understanding the impact of these lifestyle changes on blood pressure can motivate individuals to adopt healthier habits for better long-term health outcomes.

Lastly, psychological factors such as stress and anxiety can adversely affect blood pressure. Chronic stress can lead to temporary spikes in blood pressure, which may eventually contribute to hypertension. Learning stress management techniques, such as mindfulness and relaxation exercises, can aid in controlling blood pressure levels. By addressing both physical and psychological factors, individuals can take comprehensive steps towards managing their blood pressure effectively and improving their overall well-being.

9

Chapter 9: The Connection Between Sleep Apnoea and Hypertension

Defining Sleep Apnoea

Sleep apnoea is a serious sleep disorder characterised by repeated interruptions in breathing during sleep. These interruptions can last for a few seconds to minutes and may occur numerous times throughout the night. Individuals suffering from this condition often experience excessive daytime sleepiness, loud snoring, and may struggle to concentrate or function effectively during waking hours. Understanding sleep apnoea is crucial, especially as it is increasingly linked to various health issues, including high blood pressure.

The mechanisms through which sleep apnoea impacts blood pressure are complex. When breathing halts during sleep, the body reacts by becoming stressed, leading to increased production of stress hormones. This stress response can elevate blood pressure levels, creating a cycle where high blood pressure exacerbates the severity of sleep apnoea. Those who suffer from both conditions may find it particularly challenging to manage their hypertension effectively, making awareness and early diagnosis essential.

There are different types of sleep apnoea, with obstructive sleep apnoea being the most common. This type occurs when the muscles at the back of the throat relax excessively, obstructing the airway and interrupting normal breathing patterns. Central sleep apnoea, on the other hand, is caused by a failure of the brain to signal the muscles to breathe. Understanding these distinctions is vital, as the treatment approaches can vary significantly between the types, and addressing both sleep apnoea and hypertension may require a multifaceted strategy.

Management of sleep apnoea can lead to significant improvements in overall health and well-being. Lifestyle changes, such as weight loss, regular physical activity, and dietary modifications, are often recommended. In some cases, continuous positive airway pressure (CPAP) therapy may be necessary to keep the airway open during sleep. Treating sleep apnoea not only enhances sleep quality but can also contribute to better blood pressure control, ultimately reducing the risks associated with hypertension.

In summary, defining sleep apnoea highlights its critical role in understanding hypertension. As the links between these two conditions become clearer, increased awareness and education are essential for both patients and healthcare providers. Recognising the signs of sleep apnoea and seeking appropriate treatment can lead to improved health outcomes, particularly for those managing high blood pressure, thus underscoring the importance of a holistic approach to health.

Mechanisms Linking Sleep Apnoea and Hypertension

Sleep apnoea is a condition characterised by repeated interruptions in breathing during sleep, which can lead to significant health complications, including hypertension. The relationship between sleep apnoea and high blood pressure is complex and multifaceted. Individuals suffering from sleep apnoea often experience a number of physiological changes during the night, such as increased sympathetic nervous system activity, which can elevate blood pressure levels. This persistent increase in blood pressure can contribute to the development of hypertension over time, making it crucial to understand how these two conditions are interlinked.

One of the primary mechanisms linking sleep apnoea and hypertension is the intermittent hypoxia that occurs during apnoeic episodes. When a person with sleep apnoea stops breathing, oxygen levels in the blood drop significantly, prompting the body to react with a stress response. This response includes the release of stress hormones such as adrenaline, which can increase heart rate and vascular resistance, ultimately leading to elevated blood pressure. Therefore, the repeated cycles of hypoxia and reoxygenation can have a detrimental effect on cardiovascular health.

Furthermore, sleep apnoea can lead to increased inflammation within the body, another contributing factor to hypertension. Chronic inflammation is known to disrupt the normal functioning of blood vessels, making them stiffer and less capable of dilating properly. This stiffness can cause a rise in blood pressure, creating a vicious cycle where hypertension exacerbates the severity of sleep apnoea. Understanding this inflammatory link provides valuable insight into potential therapeutic approaches for managing both conditions.

Lifestyle factors, such as obesity, also play a significant role in the connection between sleep apnoea and hypertension. Excess weight can contribute to the development of sleep apnoea, as it may lead to fat accumulation around the neck and throat, increasing the likelihood of airway obstruction during sleep. This, in turn, can exacerbate hypertension, creating a challenging situation for individuals trying to manage either condition. Addressing lifestyle changes, including diet and physical activity, becomes essential for breaking this cycle.

Finally, recognising the interplay between sleep apnoea and hypertension is vital for effective management strategies. Healthcare professionals should consider screening for sleep apnoea in patients diagnosed with hypertension and vice versa. Managing sleep apnoea through various interventions, including continuous positive airway pressure (CPAP) therapy and lifestyle modifications, can significantly improve blood pressure control. Thus, understanding these mechanisms not only aids in better management of hypertension but also enhances overall cardiovascular health.

Diagnosis and Treatment Options

Diagnosing hypertension can be a complex process, as it often requires multiple readings taken over time to confirm elevated blood pressure levels. Healthcare professionals typically utilise a sphygmomanometer to measure blood pressure in millimetres of mercury (mmHg). A diagnosis of hypertension is generally made when the systolic pressure is consistently at or above 130 mmHg, or the diastolic pressure is at or above 80 mmHg. It is essential for individuals to understand that hypertension is often asymptomatic, making regular monitoring critical for early detection and management.

Once diagnosed, treatment options for hypertension can vary significantly based on individual health profiles and the severity of the condition. Lifestyle modifications are often the first line of defence and may include dietary changes such as adopting the DASH diet, which emphasises fruits, vegetables, and low-fat dairy. Additionally, reducing sodium intake and increasing physical activity can play vital roles in controlling blood pressure. For some individuals, these changes alone may be sufficient to manage their hypertension effectively.

In cases where lifestyle changes are inadequate, pharmacological treatments may be necessary. There are several classes of medications available, such as diuretics, ACE inhibitors, and calcium channel blockers, each with their own mechanisms of action and potential side effects. It is crucial for patients to have a detailed discussion with their healthcare providers about the risks and benefits of these medications, as well as any possible interactions with other drugs they may be taking. Understanding these factors can help in making informed decisions about one's treatment plan.

Moreover, the role of psychological factors cannot be overlooked in the management of hypertension. Stress management techniques, such as mindfulness and cognitive behavioural therapy, can be effective adjuncts to traditional treatment methods. Additionally, ensuring adequate sleep and addressing issues like sleep apnoea can significantly impact blood pressure levels. Patients should be encouraged to explore these avenues, as they may provide both physical and emotional benefits in the management of their condition.

Finally, regular monitoring of blood pressure is essential, whether through home devices or during clinical visits. Home monitoring can empower patients to take an active role in their health, while clinical measurements offer a professional assessment. Understanding the nuances between these methods, including their advantages and limitations, can significantly enhance an individual's ability to manage hypertension effectively. By combining lifestyle changes, medications, and psychological support, individuals can work towards achieving optimal blood pressure control and enhancing their overall health.

Lifestyle Changes to Improve Sleep Quality

Achieving quality sleep is crucial for overall health, particularly for individuals managing high blood pressure. One of the first lifestyle changes to consider is establishing a consistent sleep routine. Going to bed and waking up at the same time every day helps regulate the body's internal clock, making it easier to fall asleep and wake up refreshed. This routine can also enhance the quality of sleep, reducing the likelihood of disturbances throughout the night.

Diet plays a significant role in sleep quality as well. Consuming a balanced diet rich in fruits, vegetables, whole grains, and lean proteins can promote better sleep. Foods high in magnesium, such as nuts and leafy greens, are particularly beneficial. It is also advisable to limit caffeine and alcohol intake, especially in the hours leading up to bedtime, as these substances can interfere with sleep patterns and exacerbate hypertension.

Physical activity is another critical factor in improving sleep quality. Regular exercise not only helps control blood pressure but also promotes better sleep. Engaging in moderate physical activity, such as walking or cycling, for at least 30 minutes most days can help individuals fall asleep faster and enjoy deeper sleep. However, it is essential to avoid vigorous exercise close to bedtime, as this can have the opposite effect.

Creating a sleep-conducive environment is vital for achieving restful sleep. This includes making the bedroom dark, quiet, and cool. Investing in a comfortable mattress and pillows can also make a significant difference. Additionally, incorporating relaxation techniques such as meditation or deep breathing exercises before bedtime can help ease the mind and prepare the body for sleep, further enhancing overall sleep quality.

Finally, managing stress levels is crucial for sleep quality. Chronic stress can lead to insomnia and other sleep disorders, which may exacerbate hypertension. Practising stress-reduction techniques, such as yoga or mindfulness, can be beneficial. By adopting these lifestyle changes, individuals can not only improve their sleep quality but also take important steps towards better managing their blood pressure and overall health.

10

Chapter 10: Hypertension in Pregnancy: Risks and Management Strategies

Understanding Hypertensive Disorders in Pregnancy

Hypertensive disorders in pregnancy, including gestational hypertension and pre-eclampsia, are significant health concerns that can affect both the mother and the developing fetus. These conditions typically arise after the 20th week of gestation and are characterised by elevated blood pressure and, in some cases, the presence of protein in the urine. Understanding these disorders is crucial as they can lead to serious complications if not managed appropriately, including placental abruption, premature birth, and even maternal and infant mortality.

The underlying mechanisms of hypertensive disorders in pregnancy are complex and multifactorial. Factors such as genetics, pre-existing health conditions, and lifestyle choices, including diet and physical activity, all play a role. Women with a history of hypertension or those who are overweight are at a higher risk of developing these disorders. Therefore, it is essential for pregnant women to monitor their blood pressure regularly and consult healthcare providers for proper evaluation and management strategies.

Dietary approaches can significantly impact blood pressure control during pregnancy. Consuming a balanced diet rich in fruits, vegetables, whole grains, and lean proteins while limiting salt and processed foods can help manage hypertension. Additionally, adequate hydration and maintaining a healthy weight are vital components of a dietary strategy that supports both maternal and fetal health. Mothers-to-be should work with healthcare professionals to develop a suitable nutritional plan tailored to their needs.

Physical activity also plays a pivotal role in managing blood pressure during pregnancy. Engaging in regular, moderate exercise can help improve cardiovascular health and reduce stress levels, which are beneficial for managing hypertension. Activities such as walking, swimming, and prenatal yoga can be particularly advantageous. However, it is important for pregnant women to consult their healthcare providers before starting any new exercise regimen to ensure safety and appropriateness based on their individual health status.

Lastly, psychological factors cannot be overlooked when addressing hypertensive disorders in pregnancy. Stress management techniques, such as mindfulness and relaxation exercises, can aid in mitigating anxiety and promoting mental well-being. The interplay between psychological health and blood pressure highlights the importance of a holistic approach to pregnancy care, encompassing physical, dietary, and emotional support to ensure the best outcomes for both mother and child.

Risks to Mother and Baby

High blood pressure during pregnancy poses significant risks to both the mother and the baby. It can lead to serious complications such as preeclampsia, which affects the mother's organs and can result in premature delivery. High blood pressure may also restrict blood flow to the placenta, impacting the baby's growth and development. Therefore, understanding and managing hypertension during pregnancy is crucial for ensuring the health of both the mother and her child.

One of the primary risks associated with high blood pressure in pregnancy is the development of gestational hypertension or preeclampsia. This condition can occur after the 20th week of pregnancy and can lead to increased swelling, protein in the urine, and elevated blood pressure. If left untreated, it can escalate to eclampsia, which can cause seizures and significantly endanger both the mother and baby. Regular monitoring and early intervention are essential to mitigate these risks.

The effects of hypertension are not limited to the immediate complications during pregnancy; they can have long-term consequences as well. Mothers who experience high blood pressure during pregnancy are at a higher risk of developing cardiovascular diseases later in life. For babies, the risks include low birth weight, premature birth, and developmental issues. It is paramount for expectant mothers to engage in regular prenatal check-ups to monitor blood pressure and overall health.

Dietary approaches and lifestyle changes play a critical role in managing hypertension in pregnant women. Incorporating a balanced diet rich in fruits, vegetables, and whole grains, while reducing sodium intake, can help control blood pressure levels. Physical activity, under the guidance of a healthcare provider, can also be beneficial. These strategies not only assist in managing hypertension but also contribute to better overall health during pregnancy.

In conclusion, the risks associated with high blood pressure during pregnancy necessitate careful attention and proactive management. By understanding these risks and engaging in healthy lifestyle choices, mothers can significantly improve their chances of a safe pregnancy and a healthy baby. Continuous education on hypertension and its implications is essential for both healthcare providers and expectant mothers alike.

Management Strategies During Pregnancy

Pregnancy is a unique period that requires careful management of health, particularly for women with hypertension. High blood pressure during pregnancy can pose significant risks to both the mother and the developing fetus. Therefore, it is essential to adopt effective management strategies to ensure a healthy pregnancy outcome. This includes regular monitoring of blood pressure, consultation with healthcare providers, and adjustments to lifestyle and medication as necessary.

Dietary approaches play a crucial role in managing hypertension during pregnancy. Women are encouraged to follow a balanced diet rich in fruits, vegetables, whole grains, and lean proteins while limiting salt intake. Staying hydrated and maintaining a healthy weight can also contribute to blood pressure control. Additionally, some studies suggest that specific nutrients, such as potassium and magnesium, may help in managing hypertension and supporting overall maternal health.

Physical activity is another vital component of effective management strategies. Engaging in moderate exercise, as advised by healthcare professionals, can help in maintaining a healthy weight and reducing stress levels. Activities such as walking, swimming, or prenatal yoga are often recommended, as they can enhance cardiovascular health without putting undue strain on the body. However, it is crucial for pregnant women to consult their healthcare providers before starting any exercise regimen.

Psychological factors also significantly influence blood pressure during pregnancy. Stress management techniques, such as mindfulness, meditation, and deep-breathing exercises, can help alleviate anxiety and promote relaxation. Creating a supportive environment and seeking help from mental health professionals when needed can further contribute to better health outcomes for both the mother and the baby.

Lastly, understanding the importance of medication management is essential for women who have pre-existing hypertension or develop it during pregnancy. Healthcare providers must carefully assess the risks and benefits of antihypertensive medications, as some may not be safe during pregnancy. Regular follow-ups and open communication with healthcare professionals can ensure that any necessary adjustments are made promptly, contributing to a healthier pregnancy and reducing the risk of complications.

Postpartum Considerations

Postpartum considerations are crucial for new mothers, especially those who have experienced hypertension during pregnancy. After childbirth, women may face a range of physical and emotional challenges that can impact their overall health. Understanding how to manage blood pressure in the postpartum period is essential for ensuring long-term health and well-being. It is important for new mothers to monitor their blood pressure regularly and seek medical advice if they notice any concerning changes.

Dietary approaches play a significant role in managing hypertension after giving birth. New mothers should focus on a balanced diet rich in fruits, vegetables, whole grains, and lean proteins. Reducing salt intake and avoiding processed foods can also help maintain healthy blood pressure levels. Additionally, hydration is vital, as it supports recovery and can positively influence blood pressure regulation.

Physical activity is another important factor in postpartum hypertension management. Engaging in regular exercise can help lower blood pressure, improve mood, and aid in weight management. New mothers are encouraged to gradually incorporate physical activity into their daily routines, starting with gentle exercises and progressing as their bodies heal. Activities such as walking with the baby or participating in postnatal exercise classes can be both beneficial and enjoyable.

Psychological factors, including stress and anxiety, can significantly impact blood pressure during the postpartum period. It is essential for new mothers to recognise and address these emotional challenges. Seeking support from family, friends, or professional counselling can help alleviate stress. Mindfulness practices, such as meditation or yoga, can also be effective in managing psychological well-being and promoting a healthier lifestyle.

Finally, it is crucial to understand the potential risks associated with postpartum hypertension. Women who have experienced high blood pressure during pregnancy may be at a higher risk for developing chronic hypertension later in life. Regular check-ups with healthcare providers are necessary to monitor blood pressure levels and discuss any concerns. By taking proactive steps in diet, exercise, and mental health, new mothers can effectively manage their blood pressure and enhance their overall quality of life in the postpartum phase.

11

1. Introduction to Hypertension

Hypertension, or high blood pressure, is defined as the **force exerted by circulating blood on the walls of blood vessels**, measured in millimeters of mercury (mmHg). It is recorded with two numbers: **systolic pressure** (the higher number, measuring pressure when the heart beats) and **diastolic pressure** (the lower number, measuring pressure between heartbeats). Regular monitoring is "crucial, as they reflect the state of cardiovascular health and the efficiency of the circulatory system." Hypertension is often called the **'silent killer'** because it "frequently presents no symptoms, yet it can lead to severe health complications, including heart disease, stroke, and kidney failure."

Types of Hypertension:

- **Essential Hypertension (Primary Hypertension):** Accounts for the majority of cases and "does not have a specific identifiable cause." It is influenced by a "combination of genetic, environmental, and lifestyle factors" and often "develops gradually over many years."
- **Secondary Hypertension:** "Caused by an underlying medical condition." This type "can arise from various factors, including kidney disease, hormonal disorders, or the use of certain medications." It "can often be treated by addressing the underlying issue."

Causes and Risk Factors:

- **Genetics:** Individuals with a family history are more prone.
- **Age:** Likelihood increases with age, "particularly in individuals over the age of 45."
- **Lifestyle Factors:** Poor diet, lack of physical activity, and stress are significant contributors.

Symptoms and Diagnosis:

- **Essential Hypertension:** Often asymptomatic, hence the 'silent killer' moniker. Some may experience "vague signs such as headaches, dizziness, or shortness of breath during physical exertion." Diagnosis involves "multiple blood pressure readings taken on different occasions."
- **Secondary Hypertension:** Can appear suddenly. Symptoms may include "severe or frequent headaches," "shortness of breath, fatigue, and visual changes." Diagnosis involves "a comprehensive assessment that includes a detailed medical history and physical examination," often with "blood and urine tests" and "imaging studies."
- **When to Suspect Secondary Hypertension:** Suspect when "standard treatment methods fail to yield the expected results," "sudden onset of high blood pressure in an individual with previously normal readings," "resistant hypertension," or "hypertension occurring at a younger age than typical." Common associated conditions include "renal disease, endocrine disorders, and certain medications."

Complications of Untreated Hypertension:

Untreated hypertension can lead to severe damage across multiple body systems:

- **Cardiovascular System:** "Significantly increasing the risk of heart disease and stroke." Leads to **atherosclerosis** (artery thickening and hardening), impairing blood flow.

- **Kidneys:** Damages blood vessels in the kidneys, leading to "kidney disease or even kidney failure," potentially requiring dialysis or transplant.
- **Brain:** Can cause "cognitive decline and an increased risk of dementia" (vascular dementia) and increases stroke risk.
- **Eyes:** Can lead to **hypertensive retinopathy** (damage to retinal blood vessels), "potentially leading to vision loss" and irreversible damage.
- **Mental Health:** Can contribute to "anxiety and depression."

12

2. Management Strategies: A Holistic Approach

Effective hypertension management requires a **multifaceted, holistic approach** integrating lifestyle modifications, medical interventions, and psychological support.

2.1. Dietary Approaches

Diet plays a "pivotal role in managing hypertension."

- **The DASH Diet (Dietary Approaches to Stop Hypertension):** "Specifically designed to combat high blood pressure."
- **Principles:** Focuses on "consuming a balanced diet rich in fruits, vegetables, whole grains, and lean proteins while reducing the intake of saturated fats, cholesterol, and sodium."
- **Sodium Reduction:** Recommends limiting sodium to "no more than 2,300 milligrams per day, with an ideal goal of 1,500 milligrams for individuals with hypertension." Achieved by "avoiding processed foods, reading labels carefully, and opting for fresh ingredients." "Even a modest reduction in sodium intake can lead to noticeable improvements."
- **Potassium-Rich Foods:** Encourages "an increase in potassium-rich

foods" (e.g., bananas, spinach, sweet potatoes) to "balance the effects of sodium."

- **Low-Fat Dairy:** Promotes consumption for calcium and vitamin D.
- **Benefits:** Beyond blood pressure control, it can lead to "weight loss, improved cholesterol levels, and reduced risk of heart disease."
- **Foods to Embrace:Potassium-rich foods:** "bananas, oranges, and leafy greens."
- **Whole grains, lean proteins, healthy fats:** "nuts and avocados."
- **Fruits and vegetables:** Berries (antioxidants), beets (nitrates for vessel dilation).
- **Foods to Avoid:Processed foods:** High in sodium (canned soups, deli meats, frozen dinners).
- **Sugary beverages and excessive alcohol.**
- **Meal Planning and Preparation:**Aim for "at least five servings of fruits and vegetables each day."
- Choose "whole grains over refined grains" (brown rice, quinoa, whole grain bread).
- Use "herbs and spices to enhance flavour instead of salt."
- Incorporate "lean proteins" (skinless poultry, fish, legumes, low-fat dairy).
- Prefer cooking methods like "steaming, grilling, or baking."
- "Preparing meals at home allows for better control over ingredients."

2.2. Physical Activity

Regular exercise is a "critical factor" and "cornerstone of hypertension management."

- **Guidelines:** "At least 150 minutes a week" of "moderate-intensity activities such as brisk walking, cycling, or swimming."
- **Types of Beneficial Exercises:Aerobic exercises:** "walking, jogging, cycling, and swimming."
- **Strength training:** "resistance exercises, such as weight lifting or body-

weight workouts, at least twice a week."

- **Flexibility and balance exercises:** "yoga and tai chi" for relaxation and stress reduction.
- **Low-impact exercises:** "walking or water aerobics" are advisable for older adults.
- **Impact of Regular Exercise:** "Leads to reductions in systolic and diastolic blood pressure."
- "Promotes better blood flow, reduces arterial stiffness, and enhances the body's ability to regulate blood pressure."
- Aids in **weight management**, which "places additional strain on the heart and blood vessels."
- "Reduces stress and anxiety levels," acting as a "natural stress reliever."
- **Developing an Exercise Routine:** Start gradually with "low-impact activities."
- "Consistency is key."
- Include strength training.
- "Tracking progress through a journal or app."
- "Consulting healthcare professionals before beginning a new exercise regimen is advisable."

2.3. Psychological Factors and Stress Management

"Psychological factors... are closely linked to blood pressure changes." Chronic stress "can lead to behaviours that exacerbate hypertension."

- **Link Between Mental Health and Blood Pressure:** Stress and anxiety trigger release of "adrenaline and cortisol," temporarily increasing heart rate and blood pressure, leading to "sustained elevations" if chronic.
- Depression and anxiety "can exacerbate high blood pressure, creating a vicious cycle."
- Mental health impacts adherence to treatment and motivation for healthy habits.
- Poor sleep quality "can lead to increased stress and anxiety, which in turn

may elevate blood pressure."

- **Identifying Sources of Stress:** Common stressors include "work-related pressures, personal relationships, and financial concerns."
- **Long-term Effects of Chronic Stress:** "Increased heart rates, elevated blood pressure, and a surge in stress hormones." Can lead to hypertension, heart disease, and stroke.
- **Stress Management Techniques:Mindfulness and Meditation:** "Focus on the present moment... decrease stress hormones and promote a sense of calm."
- **Deep Breathing Exercises:** Promote relaxation.
- **Cognitive Behavioral Therapy (CBT):** Provides tools to cope effectively.
- **Relaxation Techniques:** Progressive muscle relaxation.
- **Physical Activity:** "Reduces stress levels and improves mental well-being."
- **Social Support:** "Connecting with friends and family."
- **Good Sleep Hygiene:** "Prioritising sleep is crucial."

2.4. Medications for Hypertension

Medications are often "a cornerstone in the treatment of high blood pressure," particularly when lifestyle changes are insufficient.

- **Overview:** Designed to "lower blood pressure and reduce the risk of complications such as heart attacks and strokes."
- **Common Classes of Medications:Diuretics ("water pills"):** "Help eliminate excess fluid and sodium from the body," reducing blood volume. Types: thiazide (first line), loop, potassium-sparing. Side effects: dehydration, electrolyte imbalances.
- **ACE Inhibitors & Angiotensin II Receptor Blockers (ARBs):** "Relax blood vessels" by targeting the renin-angiotensin-aldosterone system (RAAS). ACE inhibitors prevent narrowing; ARBs block action of angiotensin II. Provide "protective benefits for the heart and kidneys." Side effects: persistent cough (ACE inhibitors), dizziness, changes in kidney function.

- **Calcium Channel Blockers (CCBs):** "Reduce vascular resistance" by inhibiting calcium influx into blood vessel cells, causing relaxation and dilation. Can be beneficial for angina or arrhythmias. Side effects: swelling in legs, dizziness, flushing.
- **Beta Blockers:** "Slow heart rate and reduce cardiac output" by blocking adrenaline effects. Beneficial for stress-related hypertension. Side effects: fatigue, cold extremities, sometimes depression.
- **Alpha Blockers (Centrally Acting Agents):** Work by "blocking alpha-adrenergic receptors in the central nervous system," leading to decreased peripheral vascular resistance. Can be effective for hypertension with benign prostatic hyperplasia (BPH). Side effects: dizziness, fatigue, headaches.
- **Direct Vasodilators (for resistant cases):** Directly relax smooth muscles in blood vessel walls. Examples: hydralazine, minoxidil. Used when other treatments fail. Require careful monitoring due to side effects like reflex tachycardia and fluid retention, often needing concurrent diuretics and beta-blockers.
- **Combination Therapy:** "Often necessary due to the complex nature of blood pressure regulation." "Utilising a combination of therapies can enhance effectiveness and cater to individual needs."
- **Side Effects and Considerations:** All medications have potential side effects. Open communication with healthcare providers is crucial to manage them and discuss alternatives.
- **Adherence to Medication Regimen:** "Crucial for individuals managing high blood pressure." Factors influencing adherence include "side effects, the complexity of the dosing schedule, and a lack of understanding." Education, support systems, and self-monitoring help improve adherence.

13

3. Monitoring Blood Pressure

"Regular monitoring of blood pressure is essential for everyone," especially those at risk or diagnosed with hypertension, as it "often presents no symptoms."

Importance of Regular Monitoring:

- **Early Detection:** Helps identify abnormalities early.
- **Guiding Lifestyle Choices:** Allows individuals to see how dietary and exercise changes impact their readings.
- **Assessing Treatment Effectiveness:** Helps track how medications are working and guides adjustments.
- **Understanding Psychological Impact:** Helps recognize how stress affects blood pressure.
- **Older Adults:** "Particularly crucial due to the increased risk associated with age."

Types of Monitoring Devices:

- **Sphygmomanometer:** Manual (requires skill) or digital (automatic, common for home use).
- **Wrist Blood Pressure Monitor:** Compact and portable, but "may be less

accurate than upper arm monitors."

- **Ambulatory Blood Pressure Monitors:** Worn for 24 hours, providing "a comprehensive overview of blood pressure fluctuations throughout daily activities," useful for diagnosing "white coat hypertension."
- **Smart Monitors:** Connect to smartphones, track data, set reminders, and share results.

How to Accurately Measure Blood Pressure at Home:

1. **Choose a validated automatic digital monitor.**
2. **Prepare:** Sit quietly for a few minutes, back supported, feet flat, arm at heart level, cuff correctly placed.
3. **Consistency:** Measure at the same time daily.
4. **Avoid:** Caffeine, exercise, smoking for 30 minutes prior.
5. **Measure:** Take 2-3 readings, waiting a minute between each.
6. **Record results.**
7. **Consult healthcare provider:** Share data and discuss any significant changes. Home monitoring "does not replace regular check-ups."

Understanding Blood Pressure Readings:

- **Systolic Pressure:** Higher number, pressure when heart beats.
- **Diastolic Pressure:** Lower number, pressure between heartbeats.
- **Categories:Normal:** Around 120/80 mmHg.
- **Elevated:** 120-129 systolic and less than 80 diastolic (lifestyle changes needed).
- **Stage 1 Hypertension:** 130-139 systolic or 80-89 diastolic.
- **Stage 2 Hypertension:** 140/90 mmHg or higher.

14

4. Specific Considerations for Certain Populations

4.1. Hypertension in Older Adults

Older adults are "at a higher risk of developing hypertension" due to:

- **Age-Related Changes:** "Stiffening of blood vessels," "accumulation of plaque (atherosclerosis)," and less efficient "hormonal regulation."
- **Common Comorbidities:** Frequently coexist with hypertension, complicating management:
- **Diabetes:** Both elevate cardiovascular risk.
- **Cardiovascular Diseases:** Vicious cycle where hypertension exacerbates heart conditions.
- **Kidney Disorders:** Kidneys regulate blood pressure; impairment leads to further elevation.
- **Psychological Factors:** Depression and anxiety are common, complicating treatment.
- **Management Strategies:**Regular monitoring.
- Focus on medication adherence.
- Healthcare providers must "customise treatment plans" considering

unique health needs, potential medication side effects, and comorbidities.

- Lifestyle modifications are crucial, but exercise regimens may need to be tailored (e.g., low-impact activities).

4.2. The Connection Between Sleep Apnoea and Hypertension

"Sleep apnoea is a serious sleep disorder characterised by repeated interruptions in breathing during sleep." It is "increasingly linked to various health issues, including high blood pressure."

- **Defining Sleep Apnoea:Obstructive Sleep Apnoea (OSA):** Most common; throat muscles relax, obstructing airway.
- **Central Sleep Apnoea:** Brain fails to signal breathing muscles.
- **Mechanisms Linking Sleep Apnoea and Hypertension:Stress Response:** Breathing interruptions lead to "increased production of stress hormones," elevating blood pressure.
- **Intermittent Hypoxia:** Low oxygen levels during episodes trigger a "stress response" (adrenaline release, increased heart rate/vascular resistance).
- **Increased Inflammation:** Chronic inflammation "disrupt[s] the normal functioning of blood vessels," making them stiffer.
- **Obesity:** Excess weight contributes to both conditions, creating a vicious cycle.
- **Diagnosis and Treatment:**Screening for sleep apnoea in hypertension patients (and vice versa) is crucial.
- Treatment improves blood pressure control.
- **Lifestyle changes:** "Weight loss, regular physical activity, and dietary modifications."
- **CPAP therapy:** "Continuous positive airway pressure (CPAP) therapy may be necessary to keep the airway open."
- **Lifestyle Changes to Improve Sleep Quality:Consistent sleep routine:** Go to bed and wake up at the same time daily.
- **Diet:** Balanced diet, magnesium-rich foods; limit caffeine and alcohol before bed.

- **Physical Activity:** Regular moderate exercise (avoid vigorous activity close to bedtime).
- **Sleep-conducive environment:** Dark, quiet, cool bedroom; comfortable mattress/pillows.
- **Stress Management:** Yoga, mindfulness.

4.3. Hypertension in Pregnancy

"Significant health concerns that can affect both the mother and the developing fetus."

- **Hypertensive Disorders in Pregnancy:Gestational Hypertension:** Elevated blood pressure after 20 weeks.
- **Pre-eclampsia:** Elevated blood pressure with protein in urine.
- **Eclampsia:** Untreated pre-eclampsia leading to seizures.
- **Risks to Mother and Baby:Mother:** "Preeclampsia," organ damage, premature delivery, increased long-term risk of cardiovascular disease.
- **Baby:** Restricted blood flow to placenta, low birth weight, premature birth, developmental issues.
- **Management Strategies During Pregnancy:Regular monitoring and consultation with healthcare providers.**
- **Dietary Approaches:** Balanced diet (fruits, vegetables, whole grains, lean proteins), limit salt/processed foods, adequate hydration, healthy weight.
- **Physical Activity:** Regular, moderate exercise (walking, swimming, prenatal yoga) as advised by a healthcare provider.
- **Psychological Factors:** Stress management techniques (mindfulness, meditation), supportive environment.
- **Medication Management:** Careful assessment of risks/benefits; some antihypertensive medications are unsafe during pregnancy. Regular follow-ups essential.
- **Postpartum Considerations:**Continue "regular monitoring of blood pressure."
- **Dietary Approaches:** Balanced diet, reduce salt, avoid processed foods,

hydration.

- **Physical Activity:** Gradual incorporation of exercise (walking with baby, postnatal classes).
- **Psychological Factors:** Address stress/anxiety (family/friend support, professional counseling, mindfulness).
- **Long-term Risk:** Women with pregnancy-induced hypertension have a higher risk of chronic hypertension later in life.

15

FAQ

What is hypertension, and why is it called the "silent killer"?

Hypertension, commonly known as high blood pressure, is a condition where the force of circulating blood against the walls of blood vessels is consistently too high. It is measured in millimeters of mercury (mmHg) and expressed as two numbers: systolic pressure (when the heart beats) and diastolic pressure (between heartbeats). Hypertension is often termed the "silent killer" because it frequently presents no noticeable symptoms, yet it can lead to severe health complications over time, including heart disease, stroke, and kidney failure. Regular monitoring is crucial for early detection and management.

What are the main differences between essential and secondary hypertension?

Hypertension is primarily categorized into two types: essential and secondary. Essential hypertension, which accounts for the majority of cases, does not have a specific identifiable cause and is influenced by a combination of genetic, environmental, and lifestyle factors. It typically develops gradually over many years. In contrast, secondary hypertension is caused by an underlying medical condition, such as kidney disease, hormonal disorders, or certain medications. Unlike essential hypertension, secondary hypertension can often be be resolved by treating the underlying issue. Understanding this distinction is vital for effective diagnosis and treatment strategies.

How do diet and physical activity contribute to managing hypertension?

Dietary approaches and physical activity are critical for managing hypertension. A balanced diet rich in fruits, vegetables, whole grains, and low-fat dairy, while significantly reducing sodium intake, can lower blood pressure. The DASH (Dietary Approaches to Stop Hypertension) diet is highly recommended for its effectiveness in this regard. Regular physical activity, including aerobic exercises like walking, cycling, or swimming, strengthens the heart, improves blood circulation, and reduces both systolic and diastolic pressures. Exercise also aids in weight management, which is crucial as excess weight strains the cardiovascular system. Combining these lifestyle modifications enhances overall cardiovascular health and helps control blood pressure.

What are the serious complications of untreated hypertension?

Untreated hypertension can lead to a myriad of severe complications, primarily affecting the cardiovascular system. It significantly increases the risk of heart disease and stroke, as sustained high pressure can cause arteries to thicken and harden (atherosclerosis), impairing blood flow. Kidneys are also vulnerable, with chronic high blood pressure damaging their blood vessels, potentially leading to kidney disease or failure. The brain can suffer from reduced blood flow, leading to cognitive decline, vascular dementia, and an increased risk of strokes. Additionally, the eyes can be affected, leading to hypertensive retinopathy and potential vision loss, while mental health can decline, contributing to anxiety and depression.

What is the connection between mental health factors, such as stress, and blood pressure?

Mental health factors, especially stress and anxiety, are intricately linked to blood pressure changes and can contribute to hypertension. When stressed, the body releases hormones like adrenaline and cortisol, which temporarily increase heart rate and blood pressure. Chronic stress can lead to sustained high levels of these hormones, contributing to hypertension and exacerbating existing high blood pressure. Stress can also lead to unhealthy coping mechanisms like poor eating habits and inactivity, further impacting blood pressure. Adopting stress management techniques such as mindfulness, meditation, and regular physical activity is essential for maintaining healthy blood pressure levels and improving overall well-being.

What are the different classes of medications used to treat hypertension, and how do they work?

Several classes of medications are used to treat hypertension, each with distinct mechanisms:

- **Diuretics:** These "water pills" help the body eliminate excess sodium and water, reducing blood volume and subsequently lowering blood pressure.
- **ACE Inhibitors & ARBs (Angiotensin Receptor Blockers):** These medications relax blood vessels by targeting the renin-angiotensin-aldosterone system (RAAS). ACE inhibitors prevent the formation of angiotensin II (a vessel constrictor), while ARBs block its action at receptor sites, leading to vessel dilation and reduced blood pressure.
- **Calcium Channel Blockers (CCBs):** CCBs reduce vascular resistance by inhibiting calcium influx into blood vessel smooth muscle cells, causing them to relax and dilate, which lowers blood pressure and reduces the heart's workload.
- **Beta Blockers:** These drugs block the effects of adrenaline on the heart, slowing the heart rate and reducing cardiac output, effectively lowering

blood pressure, especially for stress-related hypertension.

- **Alpha Blockers:** These centrally acting agents block alpha-adrenergic receptors, leading to decreased peripheral vascular resistance and relaxed blood vessels.
- **Direct Vasodilators:** Used for resistant cases, these medications directly relax the smooth muscles in blood vessel walls, significantly reducing vascular resistance.

Combination therapy is often needed due to the complex nature of blood pressure regulation and individual patient responses.

Why is regular blood pressure monitoring important, and what are the types of monitoring devices available?

Regular blood pressure monitoring is essential for early detection, effective management, and proactive health maintenance, especially since hypertension often presents no symptoms. Consistent monitoring helps individuals understand their cardiovascular health, assess the impact of lifestyle changes (diet, exercise), and recognize how stress affects their blood pressure.

Common monitoring devices include:

- **Manual Sphygmomanometers:** Require a stethoscope and skill for operation.
- **Automatic Digital Monitors:** Most common for home use, offering ease and storage of readings.
- **Wrist Blood Pressure Monitors:** Portable but can be less accurate than upper arm devices.
- **Ambulatory Blood Pressure Monitors:** Worn for 24 hours, providing a comprehensive overview of daily fluctuations.
- **Smart Monitors:** Connect to smartphones, allowing tracking, reminders, and sharing of data with healthcare providers.

Accurate home measurement involves proper preparation (sitting quietly, arm at heart level), correct cuff placement, and taking multiple readings at consistent times.

What is sleep apnoea, and how is it linked to hypertension?

Sleep apnoea is a serious sleep disorder characterized by repeated interruptions in breathing during sleep. These interruptions lead to significant drops in blood oxygen levels, triggering a stress response in the body. This response involves the release of stress hormones like adrenaline, which increases heart rate and vascular resistance, ultimately elevating blood pressure. The repeated cycles of oxygen deprivation and stress contribute to the development and exacerbation of hypertension. Furthermore, sleep apnoea can lead to increased inflammation and is often linked to obesity, both of which are contributing factors to high blood pressure. Addressing sleep apnoea through lifestyle changes (weight loss, physical activity) or therapies like CPAP can significantly improve blood pressure control and overall cardiovascular health.

16

📚 Books

Patient-Friendly

1. **“Mayo Clinic 5 Steps to Controlling High Blood Pressure”** – Mayo Clinic StaffA clear and practical guide with lifestyle tips and medical explanations.
2. **“The DASH Diet Action Plan”** by Marla HellerBased on NIH research, this book outlines the DASH diet in an easy-to-follow way.
3. **“Hypertension: A Companion to Braunwald’s Heart Disease”** by George L. Bakris & Matthew SorrentinoMore advanced, but has useful clinical pearls if you want depth.
4. **“Controlling High Blood Pressure the Natural Way”** by David Carroll and Wahida S. KarmallyFocuses on lifestyle management and patient empowerment.

Professional/Clinical

1. **“Hypertension: A Clinical Guide”** by Julian SeguraA practical, evidence-based clinical reference with diagnostic and therapeutic insights.
2. **“Hypertension: A Companion to Braunwald’s Heart Disease”** – a comprehensive and authoritative clinical reference.

3. **"Oxford Handbook of Hypertension"** – covers diagnosis, treatment, and management strategies.
4. **Australian Therapeutic Guidelines: Cardiovascular** – Excellent local reference with evidence-based algorithms.

17

📖 Articles & Reviews

1. **2020 ISH Global Hypertension Practice Guidelines**Link – by the International Society of Hypertension
2. **JNC 8 Guidelines for the Management of Hypertension in Adults**James PA et al. *JAMA*. 2014;311(5):507–520. [PMID: 24352797]
3. **2023 ACC/AHA Hypertension Guidelines Summary**Useful for clinicians to understand evolving targets and recommendations.
4. **"Hypertension in Adults: Screening and Diagnosis"** – *American Family Physician*, updated guideline summaries
5. **"The Global Burden of Hypertension"** – *The Lancet*, articles exploring trends, disparities, and global strategies

18

🌐 Websites

For Patients

1. **Heart Foundation (Australia)** – Blood Pressure HubAustralian resource with practical, readable advice.
2. **Better Health Channel (VicGov)**Reliable government-approved content tailored to the public.
3. **American Heart Association – High Blood Pressure**Interactive tools, videos, and diet tips.
4. **NHS UK – High Blood Pressure (Hypertension)**
5. **Centers for Disease Control and Prevention (CDC)** – HypertensionPrevention-focused, with downloadable PDFs and infographics.

For Professionals

1. **Australian Heart Foundation – Clinical Guidelines**Local recommendations, algorithms, and patient handouts.
2. **UpToDate** *(subscription required)*In-depth articles with ongoing updates, especially useful for secondary hypertension.
3. **BMJ Best Practice – Hypertension** *(subscription)*Excellent summaries with evidence grades.

4. **The Cochrane Library** – Hypertension ReviewsSystematic reviews of interventions for lifestyle, diet, and meds.